Simple Home Herbal Remedies

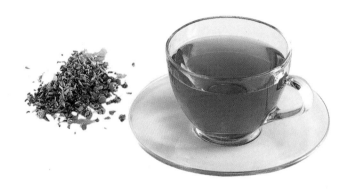

Penelope Ody

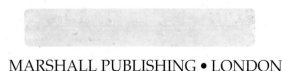

MARSHALL PUBLISHING • LONDON

A Marshall Edition
Conceived, edited and designed by
Marshall Editions
The Orangery
161 New Bond Street
London W1Y 9PA

First published in the UK in 1999 by
Marshall Publishing Ltd

ISBN: 1 84 028 300 9

Originated in Singapore by Chroma Graphics
Printed and bound in Portugal by Printer
Portuguesa

Project Editor Jo Wells

Editor Theresa Reynolds

Additional Editing Madeline Weston

Researcher Diana Walsh

Indexer Sue Cawthorne

Art Editor Siân Keogh

Designer Sandra Marques

Photographer David Jordan

Stylist Kim Davies

Picture Research Antonella Mauro

Managing Editor Anne Yelland

Managing Art Editor Helen Spencer

Editorial Director Ellen Dupont

Art Director Dave Goodman

Editorial Coordinator Becca Clunes

Production Nikki Ingram

Note

Every effort has been taken to ensure that all
information in this book is correct and
compatible with national standards generally
accepted at the time of publication. This book is
not intended to replace consultation with your
doctor or other healthcare professional. The
author and publisher disclaim any liability, loss,
injury or damage incurred as a consequence,
directly or indirectly, of the use and application
of the contents of this book.

CONTENTS

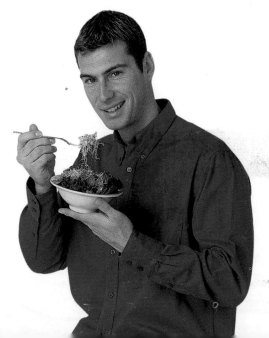

Herbs for the mind

Herbs for men and women

Herbs for children

Herbs to keep you healthy

INTRODUCTION

Interest in herbal remedies has grown steadily in recent years. The widespread availability of low-cost medical care and modern drugs helped to create a culture where many people believed doctors could provide an instant cure for all ills, but we are beginning to recognize that good health depends more on healthy living than on antibiotics.

Herbal medicine has always been a therapy of self-help: even today traditional societies pass on favourite remedies between generations. As the West rediscovers these remedies then perhaps we, too, will replace the chemicals in the first-aid box with a garden of healing plants that cure not only our physical ills but those of mind and spirit as well.

CONSULTING A HERBALIST

A professional herbalist can advise on the most appropriate home remedies and may prescribe herbs not readily available to the public. The herbalist will typically take a detailed case history and carry out routine checks. Existing orthodox medication should be discussed so that any incompatibility with herbal remedies can be taken into account. He or she will prescribe and dispense the remedy, and may also give advice on diet, relaxation or Bach Flower Remedies to treat emotional factors. Some herbalists prescribe remedies to ease symptoms, while others focus on holistic treatments involving major lifestyle changes.

QUALIFIED HERBALISTS

In Britain, members of the National Institute of Medical Herbalists qualify by examination after four years of study. Some UK universities also offer degree courses in herbal medicine. In France herbal practitioners (*phytotherapists*) are almost always trained doctors, while in Germany they have comparable status to orthodox GPs. In some countries it is illegal to prescribe herbal remedies.

Professional bodies

General Council and Register of Consultant Herbalists, Marlborough House, Swanpool, Falmouth, Cornwall TR11 4HW.

National Institute of Medical Herbalists, 56 Longbrook Street, Exeter, Devon EX4 6AH.

The Register of Chinese Herbal Medicine, PO Box 400, Wembley, Middlesex HA9 9NZ.

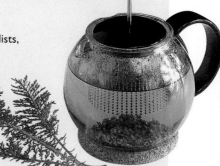

BOTANICAL NAMES OF HERBS

BOTANICAL NAME	COMMON NAME	PARTS USED
Achillea millefolium	Yarrow	Aerial parts, oil
Agathosma betulina	Buchu	Leaves
Agrimonia eupatoria	Agrimony	Aerial parts
Alchemilla xanthoclora	Lady's mantle	Aerial parts
Allium sativa	Garlic	Bulb
Aloes spp	Aloes	Liquid drained from the
(including A. vera, A. ferox,		cut leaves;
A. perryi)	Aloe vera	sap and leaves
Alpinia galanga	Galangal	Rhizomes
Althea officinale	Marshmallow	Leaves, roots
Anemopaegma arvense	Catuaba	Tree bark
Anethum graveolens	Dill	Seeds
Angelica archangelica	Angelica	Leaves, root
Angelica polyphorma var. sinensis	Chinese angelica/dang gui	Rhizome
Arctium lappa	Burdock	Leaf, root, seeds
Arnica montana	Arnica	Flowers
Artemisia absinthum	Wormwood	Leaves, juice
Asclepias tuberosa	Pleurisy root	Root
Ascophyllum nodosum	Kelp	Seaweed
Astragalus membranaceus	Astragalus	Root
Avena sativa	Wild oats	Seeds, whole unripe plant
Ballota nigra	Black horehound	Aerial parts
Bellis perennis	Daisy	Aerial parts
Berberis vulgaris	Barberry	Stem, root, root bark
Borago officinalis	Borage	Aerial parts, seed oil
Brassica nigra	Mustard	Seed, oil
Brassica oleracea	Cabbage	Leaves
Calendula officinalis	Marigold	Petals
Capsella bursa-pastoris	Shepherd's purse	Aerial parts
Capsicum spp	Cayenne	Fruit
Carum carvi	Caraway	Oil, seeds
Centaurium erythraea	Centaury	Aerial parts
Centella asiatica	Gotu kola	Aerial parts
Chelidonium majus	Greater celandine	Aerial parts, sap
Chondrus crispus	Irish moss	Whole plant
Cimicifuga racemosa	Black cohosh	Rhizome
Citrus aurantium	Bitter orange, Neroli, Bergamot	Peel, flower oil, peel oil
Citrus limon	Lemon	Juice, oil
Cinnamonum camphora	Camphor	Crystallised distillate
		from wood
Cinnamomum zeylanicum	Cinnamon	Bark, oil
Codonopsis pilosella	Codonopsis/dang shen	Root
Commiphora myrrha	Myrrh	Oleo-gum resin
Coriandrum sativum	Coriander	Leaves, seeds
Crataegus laevigata; C. monogyna	Hawthorn	Flowers, berries
Dioscorea villosa	Wild yam	Rhizome, root
Echinacea spp	Echinacea	Root
Elettaria cardamomum	Cardamom	Seed, oil
Eleutherococcus senticosus	Siberian ginseng	Rhizome
Elymus repens	Couchgrass	Rhizome
Equisetum arvense	Horsetail	Aerial parts
Eschscholzia californica	Californian poppy	Aerial parts
Eucalyptus globulus	Eucalyptus	Leaves, oil
Eupatorium perfoliatum	Boneset	Aerial parts
Euphrasia officinalis	Eyebright	Aerial parts

BOTANICAL NAMES OF HERBS

BOTANICAL NAME	COMMON NAME	PARTS USED
Fagopyrum esculentum	Buckwheat	Aerial parts
Foeniculum vulgare	Fennel	Seeds
Forsythia suspensa	Forsythia/lian qiao	Berries
Fucus fresiculosis	Bladderwrack	Thallus
Galium aparine	Cleavers	Aerial parts
Ganoderma lucidem	Reishi	Fruiting body
Gentiana lutea	Yellow gentian	Roots, rhizomes
Geranium maculatum	American cranesbill	Aerial parts, root
Geranium robertianum	Herb Robert	Aerial parts
Ginkgo biloba	Ginkgo	Leaves
Glycyrrhiza glabra	Liquorice	Root
Guaiacum officinale	Lignum vitae	Wood raspings, resin
Hamamelis virginiana	Witch hazel	Leaves, branches, bark
Harpagophytum procumbens	Devil's claw	Tuber
Hieracium pilosella	Mouse ear	Aerial parts
Humulus lupulus	Hops	Female flowers
Hypericum perforatum	St John's wort	Herb
Hyssopus officinale	Hyssop	Aerial parts, oil
Inula helenium	Elecampane	Root, flowers
Jasminium officinale	Jasmine	Essential oil
Juniperis communis	Juniper	Berries, oils
Lactuca verosa	Wild lettuce	Leaves, dried juice
Lamium album	White deadnettle	Aerial parts
Lavandula angustifolia	Lavender	Flowers, oil
Lentinula edodes	Shiitake mushrooms	Fruiting body
Leonurus cardiaca	Motherwort	Aerial parts
Lycopus virginicus	Bugleweed	Aerial parts
Malva sylvestris	Common mallow	Aerial parts
Marrubium vulgare	White horehound	Aerial parts
Matricaria recutita	Chamomile	Flowers
Melaleuca alternifolia	Tea tree	Essential oil
Melilotis officinalis	Melilot	Aerial parts
Melissa officinalis	Lemon balm	Leaves, oil
Mentha x piperita	Peppermint	Leaves, essential oil
Menyanthes trifoliata	Bogbean	Leaves
Nepeta cataria	Catmint	Aerial parts
Ocimum basilicum	Basil	Leaves, oil
Oenothera biennis	Evening primrose	Seed oil
Origanum spp	Marjoram	Aerial parts, oil
Panax ginseng	Ginseng/Korean ginseng	Root
Panax quinquefolius	American ginseng	Roots
Passiflora incarnata	Passionflower	Aerial parts
Paullinia cupana	Guarana	Seed
Petroselinum crispum	Parsley	Leaves, seed
Pimpinella anisum	Anise	Seeds, oil
Pinus sylvestris	Pine	Essential oil
Plantago major	Common plantain	Leaves
Plantago ovata	Isphagula	Seeds
Plantago psyllium	Psyllium	Seeds
Pogostemon patchouli	Patchouli	Essential oil
Polygonun bistorta	Bistort	Root
Populus candicans	Balm of Gilead	Leaf buds
Potentilla erecta	Tormentil	Root

BOTANICAL NAMES OF HERBS

BOTANICAL NAME	COMMON NAME	PARTS USED
Primula veris	Cowslip	Root, flower
Prunus serotina	Wild cherry	Bark, fruit
Pulsatilla vulgaris	Pasque flower	Flowering plant
Quercus spp	Oak	Bark
Rhamnus frangula	Alder buckthorn	Bark
Rhamnus purshianus	Cascara sagrada	Bark
Rheum palmatum	Rhubarb	Rhizome
Ribes nigrum	Blackcurrant	Seed oil
Rosa spp	Rose	Petals, hips, oil
Rosmarinus officinalis	Rosemary	Leaves, oil
Rubus idaeus	Raspberry	Leaves, fruit
Rumex crispus	Yellow dock	Root
Salvia officinalis	Purple sage	Leaves, oil
Salix alba	White willow	Leaves, bark
Sambucus nigra	Elder	Flowers, berries, leaves, bark
Sanguinaria canadensis	Bloodroot	Root
Santalum alba	Sandalwood	Essential oil
Scrophularia ningpoensis	Chinese figwort/xuan shen	Root
Scrophularia nodosa	Figwort	Aerial parts
Scutellaria lateriflora	Skullcap	Aerial parts
Senna alexandrina	Senna	Leafs, pods
Serenoa repens	Saw palmetto	Fruits
Silybum marianum	Milk thistle	Seeds
Solidago vigaurea	Golden rod	Aerial parts
Stachys officinalis	Wood betony	Aerial parts
Stellaria media	Chickweed	Herb
Styrax benzoin	Benzoin	Gum resin
Symphytum officinalis	Comfrey	Root, leaves
Syzygium aromaticum	Cloves	Flower buds, oil
Tabebuia impetiginosa	Pau d'arco	Wood, inner bark
Taraxacum officinale	Dandelion	Root, leaves
Thuja occidentalis	Thuja	Twigs
Thymus vulgaris	Thyme	Aerial parts, oil
Tilia cordata	Lime	Flowers
Trifolium pratense	Red clover	Flowers
Trigonella foenum-graecum	Fenugreek	Seeds, aerial parts
Turnera diffusa var. aphrodisiaca	Damiana	Leaves
Tussilago farfara	Coltsfoot	Flowers, leaves
Ulmus rubra	Slippery elm	Inner bark
Uncaria tomentosa	Peruvian cat's claw	Inner bark
Urtica dioica	Stinging nettles	Aerial parts
Valeriana officinalis	Valerian	Root
Verbascum thapsus	Mullein	Leaves, flowers
Verbena officinalis	Vervain	Aerial parts
Viburnum opulus	Cramp bark	Bark
Viburnum prunifolium	Black haw	Stem and root barks
Vinca major	Periwinkle	Aerial parts
Viola odorata	Sweet violet	Aerial parts
Viola tricolor	Heartsease	Aerial parts
Withania somnifera	Winter cherry	Root
Zanthoxylum americanum	Prickly ash	Bark
Zea mays	Cornsilk	Stamens
Zingiber officinale	Ginger	Root, oil

HERBS FOR MINOR AILMENTS

Our great-grandmothers would have thought nothing odd about gathering plants from the hedgerow or garden to treat their family's minor ills. Professional physicians were an expensive rarity for most people and self-help was the accepted alternative.

Today, in contrast, we head for the doctor's surgery expecting instant cures from antibiotics and analgesics, and our home first-aid box is likely to be stocked with expensive pharmaceutical drugs.

Yet the kitchen cupboard and a basic assortment of herbal remedies can deal with the majority of minor self-limiting household ills, just as effectively and far more economically. All that is lacking are the skill and knowledge that our great-grandparents took for granted.

FIRST AID

In summer, the garden or window box can be the "herbal first-aid kit", with plenty of fresh green remedies to choose from: plantain leaves to soothe insect bites, fresh lavender flowers for headaches, or thick comfrey leaves to wrap around sprained ankles and wrists. In winter we need to resort to more conventional lotions and creams.

READY-MADE HERBAL PRODUCTS

As well as the kitchen standbys mentioned in the box below, the herbal first-aid box should include the following conventional herbal preparations to deal a wide range of minor emergencies and ailments:

■ Arnica cream for bruises and sprains – but arnica should not be used on broken skin because of its toxicity.

■ Homoeopathic arnica 6X tablets to be taken after shocks or accidents – allow one tablet to dissolve on the tongue and repeat every 30 minutes until the patient begins to feel more settled.

THE FIRST-AID BOX

As well as the usual stock of bandages and dressings, the herbal first-aid kit can include familiar kitchen ingredients such as ordinary Indian tea for diarrhoea, garlic cloves to draw corns, honey to clear pus from wounds and fresh ginger root for nausea and chills. Keep an *Aloe vera* plant, too – simply break off a leaf, split it open and apply the thick gel to minor burns, scalds, sunburn and grazes.

■ Chamomile tea bags for treating shock, nervous upsets, insomnia or indigestion.

■ Chickweed cream for drawing stubborn splinters, boils and insect stings and as a soothing treatment for irritant skin rashes.

■ Comfrey ointment or infused oil to encourage healing of wounds and bruises and as a massage for sprains and strains. Use only on clean cuts, as the rapidly healing cut may trap dirt, and avoid prolonged use on open wounds (see p.14).

■ Echinacea tablets as a herbal antibiotic for colds, influenza and other infections (see p.102).

■ Elderflower tea bags for colds and catarrh.

■ Fennel tea bags for digestive upsets including indigestion, or to use the soaked bags as pads for eyestrain and inflammations.

■ Garlic cloves or garlic-oil pearles. Rub fresh cloves on acne and pimples or to draw corns. The pearles can be taken for infections or the oil they contain used for ear problems.

■ Lavender oil ready diluted in almond oil – use 5 ml of lavender oil to 20 ml of almond oil and store in a dark glass 25 ml bottle. Use as a massage for headaches or dab on cold sores and minor burns.

■ Marigold (calendula) cream as an antiseptic for cuts and grazes, and an antifungal remedy for fungal infections such as athlete's foot.

■ Myrrh tincture to add to mouth washes and gargles for sore throats, gum problems and mouth ulcers.

■ Peppermint tea bags for indigestion and nausea.

■ Dr Bach's Rescue Remedy as an emergency treatment for shocks and nervous upsets. Take two or three drops neat on the tongue.

■ Slippery elm tablets to line the stomach and reduce inflammation in gastritis, for indigestion or to prevent hangovers.

■ Tea tree oil as an antiseptic and anti-fungal remedy for cuts and grazes, warts, fungal infections and cold sores.

■ Distilled witch hazel for use as a styptic on cuts and grazes and to soothe minor burns, sunburn, insect bites, varicose veins or bruises.

■ Vervain tea bags for infusions for stress and digestive problems.

TRAVELLER'S FIRST-AID KIT

Pack the following to deal with minor ills on holiday:

■ 5 ml of lavender oil in 20 ml of infused St. John's wort oil in a 25 ml bottle as a soothing treatment for sunburn.

■ 5 ml of melissa oil in 20 ml of almond oil in a 25 ml bottle as an insect repellent.

■ A 50 ml bottle containing equal amounts of St. John's wort and marigold tinctures – dilute in water to bathe cuts, grazes and insect bites.

■ Arnica cream for bruises.

■ A 50 ml bottle of meadowsweet tincture for stomach upsets – take in 5ml doses.

■ Black or Indian tea bags for soothing diarrhoea and hangovers.

■ Crystallized ginger to chew for travel sickness.

■ Siberian ginseng tablets to combat jet lag.

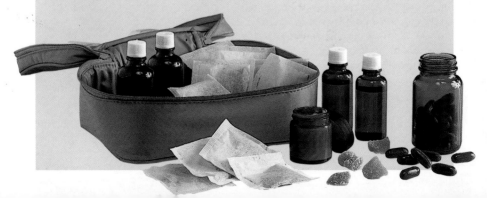

MINOR INJURIES

Herbs make useful and effective alternatives to the standard antiseptic and anti-inflammatory creams found in the family first-aid box. They can also be valuable when accidents happen far from home with only the hedgerow to turn to for immediate healing help.

BRUISES

Bruises are caused by blood escaping from damaged blood vessels just under the skin following an injury. Their multicoloured healing cycle mirrors the breakdown and dispersal of this blood.

Both arnica and comfrey will speed this healing process. Soak a clean cloth in a mixture of one teaspoon of arnica tincture in 500 ml of warm water to make a compress and apply this to new bruises. Replace the compress with a fresh hot one when it cools and repeat for as long as you can – several hours or until the pain eases. Alternatively, apply arnica or comfrey creams or infused comfrey oil every few hours, or, if you have comfrey in the garden, blend a handful of fresh leaves in a food processor and use as a poultice.

CUTS AND GRAZES

Minor cuts and grazes often need little more than bathing in warm water to clean the wound, then a herbal lotion or cream to stop bleeding, encourage healing and prevent infection. Always wash wounds from centre to edge so that any dirt is taken away from the injury. Well-strained marigold infusion makes a useful antiseptic lotion.

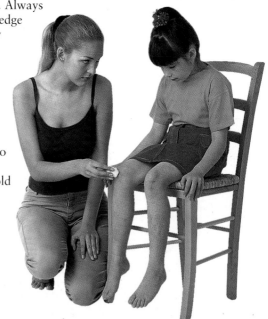

To help stop bleeding, soak a cotton swab in a cup of warm water containing one teaspoon of shepherd's purse tincture and press this to the wound for a couple of minutes. Apply a little marigold or tea tree cream as an antiseptic and cover with a suitable sticking plaster or bandage.

For minor grazes, simply smear the fresh sap from an *Aloe vera* leaf onto the wound after washing.

SPLINTERS

It is usually easy to extract splinters using a sterilized needle and tweezers but for deeply embedded ones, herbal drawing ointments may be helpful. Apply either chickweed or slippery elm ointment directly to the site of the splinter, cover with a sticking plaster and leave for at least three hours. This will usually bring the splinter to the surface where it can easily be removed. If not, clean the area and repeat using fresh ointment.

HEDGEROW HEALERS

Wild herbs can make an ideal emergency treatment when minor accidents occur on country walks or camping holidays and the first-aid box is miles away. If you're not familiar with these herbs, use a botanical field guide to ensure correct identification, and seek professional help for serious cuts, burns and sprains as soon as possible – an anti-tetanus injection may be necessary.

Herb		Action
Common mallow		Traditionally used as a substitute for marshmallow. Crush the leaves and flowers and use them as a poultice for wounds.
Plantain		Known as "white man's foot" in North America because it spread so rapidly with the settlers, can be rubbed on insect bites to relieve itching.
Daisy		Traditionally called bruisewort, will relieve bruises and sprains. Use a poultice of fresh daisies or a compress soaked in an infusion.
Yarrow		Can be used to stop nosebleeds. Use it in a fresh poultice or insert a leaf in the nostrils. Bind washed, fresh leaves to cuts and grazes.
Shepherd's purse		Can help stop bleeding – apply the leaves as a fresh poultice to cuts and grazes.
Herb Robert		Apply the fresh leaves to cuts and grazes to stop bleeding. Crush to leaves to repel mosquitoes.

ACHES AND PAINS

Injuries such as twisted ankles, sprained joints and pulled muscles are commonplace and often very painful. If the pain is acute, there are problems moving the affected joint or limb, or it seems an odd shape, then seek professional treatment without delay. The sooner broken bones are reset and torn ligaments repaired the better.

BACKACHE

The causes of an aching back can range from an excess of gardening to gynaecological problems. Persistent or chronic backache needs professional investigation. Manipulation from an osteopath or chiropractor can often be more effective than painkillers or bed rest.

MUSCLE TENSION

If back pain is associated with muscle tension, take a cup of decoction containing equal amounts of valerian and cramp bark (one teaspoon of the mix per cup) up to three times a day.

MUSCLE STRAIN

valerian

If back pain is caused by excessive exertion or obviously strained muscles (see opposite), try a long soak in a hot bath containing soothing oils; add 10 drops of rosemary,

cramp bark

juniper or thyme oil to the bath water. Then massage the aching area with a mixture of two drops of each of these oils in a teaspoon of almond oil.

COMFREY

Comfrey was once known as "knitbone", reflecting its traditional use in healing fractures. The herb contains a chemical called allantoin which encourages the growth of various tissue cells and so increases healing rates. It has had a chequered history in recent years. In the 1970s it was acclaimed as a wonder-cure for arthritis, only to be condemned in the 1980s as a source of pyrrolizidine alkaloids, which are known carcinogens. In Europe it is still acceptable as an external remedy but there is a total ban on comfrey in Australia and many American States.

While some authorities argue that the research condemning comfrey is flawed (it involved feeding large amounts of the herb to rats, who suffered from malnutrition as a result), it is best to approach the herb with caution. Do not use comfrey internally or apply it to broken skin – apart from the toxic alkaloids it contains, allantoin can speed tissue growth to such an extent that it can heal the wound before any dirt or pus has had a chance to escape.

STRAINS AND SPRAINS

A strain is when a muscle or tendon is slightly
torn, usually due to over-stretching. A sprain is a
tear in the joint capsule or its associated
ligaments, usually following a twisting injury.
  Arnica will relieve the pain, while comfrey
increases cell growth and so speeds healing. Use an
arnica compress (see Bruises, p.12) or apply a cream
or ointment containing either of these herbs. If
possible, carefully strap the injured joint with an
elastic bandage to support and compress it. Rest the
injured limb as much as possible – keep an injured
leg raised to help prevent swelling.

ACCELERATING HEALING

Alternating hot and cold treatments can bring
out any bruising and speed healing.
Depending on the site of the injury, you can
use a bowl as a foot or hand bath or apply
compresses. Make a very hot infusion of
rosemary or add one teaspoon of
rosemary oil to a bowl of hot
water. Soak your compress and
apply or place the injured limb
in this for as long as you can
bear, then transfer to a bowl of
iced water for three to four
minutes. Repeat for as long as you
can or until the symptoms start to ease.

FRACTURES

Most fractures need professional treatment with suitable splints, plaster or
support bandages, but herbs can still play their part. Broken and
cracked toes and ribs, for example, are often treated with
little more than rest and caution.

PROMOTING HEALING

Gently apply a little infused comfrey oil, a
compress soaked in comfrey infusion or
puréed fresh comfrey leaves (the purée will
set hard and form a protective green
coating) to speed up healing. Once a fracture
has been set and bandaged, take two teaspoons
of horsetail juice or a cup of horsetail decoction
three times a day; this will provide silica to
increase tissue growth and healing.

COLDS AND FLU

Antibiotics have no effect on colds and flu, as both are viral problems. Staying in bed in a warm room and drinking plenty of fluids while easing symptoms with cough mixtures and painkillers is the usual approach. Many herbs display anti-viral activity so they can be of real benefit in helping the immune system.

THE COMMON COLD

Frequent colds can be a sign of weakened immunity – related perhaps to over-exhaustion, stress or food intolerance – and some of the more powerful herbal tonics (see pp.102–105), such as astragalus, can be helpful in tackling the problem. For more general use, the most popular anti-infection herb is echinacea. Take one teaspoon of tincture or 600 mg in capsules three times a day at the first hint of a cold.

Garlic has anti-viral properties, so use plenty in cooking and take up to 1 g in capsules daily. Garlic's potent chemicals are excreted via the lungs, so it is especially useful if the cold develops into a chest infection.

A popular general-purpose tea is made with equal amounts of elder flower, yarrow and peppermint. Use one teaspoon of the mix per cup and add a pinch of cayenne while infusing the tea. Drink up to four cups daily. For the treatment of specific cold symptoms, see Sore Throat, p.40; Catarrh and sinusitis, p.36; and Coughs, p.38.

INFLUENZA

Full-blown influenza is far more unpleasant than a bad cold. Typical symptoms include the usual cold symptoms plus headaches, muscle pain, weakness and a high temperature. An attack will usually last for about a week and can leave the sufferer feeling depressed and debilitated for weeks after that.

HERBAL REMEDIES

Regular doses of echinacea are central to treatment. In addition make a tea containing equal amounts of elder flower, white horehound, yarrow and boneset (two teaspoons of the mix per cup, taken four times a day); add a pinch of powdered cinnamon to each cup. Go to bed and drink plenty of fluids – either in the form of herbal infusions or warmed fruit juices.

Severe cases

While influenza is usually unpleasant but self-limiting, it can be serious for the elderly, very young, chronically ill or for those suffering from respiratory problems, such as asthma. In such cases do not delay seeking professional help.

INHALATIONS

Steam inhalations (see p.37) can also be helpful
– put five drops each of pine, eucalyptus and
tea tree oil into a basin of boiling water.
Lean over the basin, draping a towel over
your head to trap the steam, and inhale
the fumes for as long as you can.

RECOVERY

To combat lingering depression
and chesty coughs after the
symptoms of flu have abated,
make a tea containing equal
amounts of elecampane,
vervain and St. John's
wort and drink up to
three cups daily.

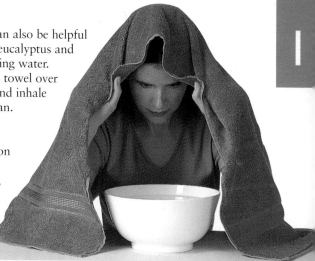

COLD SORES

Cold sores are more of a nuisance than a serious health hazard, and can
respond well to herbal remedies. The virus that causes them (*Herpes simplex*
type 1) is carried by around 50 percent of the adult population, so they're very
common. Once infected, carriers of the virus are liable to a crop of cold sores
whenever they are over-worked, run down or heading for a cold.

EARLY ACTION

Suffers from cold sores soon learn to recognize the tingling sensation that
usually occurs where a sore is about to develop. This is the best time to start
the following treatments, which may stop the sore developing entirely.

■ Apply one drop of neat tea tree oil or a 50 percent solution of
lavender, clove or melissa essential oils to the site (dilute one
teaspoon of any of these oils with one teaspoon of water),
and repeat as often as you can during the day.

■ Drink regular cups of lemon balm infusion – this herb
shows significant anti-viral activity to *Herpes simplex*.

REMEDIES

■ If a a cold sore does appear despite early
treatment, apply a little tea tree or marigold
cream while it is still at the blistering stage.

■ In addition, taking echinacea
tincture or tablets (one teaspoon
or 600 mg in capsules three times
a day) will also help to combat
any developing infections.

SKIN INFECTIONS

Minor, localized skin infections generally respond well to herbal treatments. The micro-organisms causing the problems are almost always present on our skin, but they're opportunist creatures that take advantage of any decrease in our immunity. Boils, fungal infections and warts are far more likely when we're tired or recovering from an illness. They can also suggest chronic underlying diseases, such as diabetes, so seek professional help for recurrent problems.

ACNE

Commonest during puberty due to hormonal activity, acne is generally caused by inflamed sebaceous glands and an excess of the sebum they produce. Sufferers should cut down on foods that encourage sebum production – refined carbohydrates, fried foods, animal fats, sweets and alcohol.

REMEDIES
Make an infusion from equal amounts of heartsease, nettles, burdock leaves and gotu kola (use one or two teaspoons per cup); drink three cups a day. For external use, combine 25 ml each of rosewater and distilled witch hazel with 20 drops of tea tree oil. Apply with a cotton wool swab three or more times a day.

BOILS AND CARBUNCLES

Boils are hard, inflamed, pus-filled swellings, generally caused by staphylococcal infection. A carbuncle is a cluster of boils.

TREATMENT
To burst the boil and extract the pus, apply slippery elm and marshmallow ointment, or a paste made by mixing the same powdered herbs with hot water, and cover with gauze. (If using the paste, repeat with a fresh hot poultice as the mix cools until the central core discharges.) A poultice of freshly pulped cabbage leaves is also effective. Any pus that is discharged should be carefully removed and the area bathed in an antiseptic lotion (such as dilute marigold tincture) to avoid spreading the infection.

■ Echinacea cream will help to bring the boil to a head.

■ Taking echinacea (5 ml tincture or 600 mg in capsules three times a day) will combat the infection.

ATHLETE'S FOOT AND RINGWORM

These fungal infections are caused by various species of *Tinea*, with symptoms ranging from inflammation and itching to soreness and scaling of the skin. These fungi thrive in warm, damp places so dry the skin thoroughly after bathing – especially between the toes. If the scalp is affected, avoid wearing tight hats which may encourage sweating.

REMEDIES AND PREVENTION

■ For internal treatment, take echinacea (5 ml or 600 mg three times a day) to help combat the infection and boost immunity.

■ Externally, bathe the affected areas with a lotion made by mixing 10 ml of thuja tincture in 25 ml of distilled water.

■ Apply tea tree or marigold cream to soothe dry irritated areas.

■ Sprinkle a little powdered myrrh in socks to help combat athlete's foot.

WARTS AND VERRUCAS

Warts are caused by a virus which makes the skin cells multiply abnormally to form a hard lump. They usually appear on the hands, knees and face and are mildly contagious although usually harmless. Most eventually disappear of their own accord. Verrucas or plantar warts form on the soles of the feet, where constant pressure causes them to thicken and become painful. Warts on the genitals and anus need professional treatment, as do warts that appear to erupt on the site of moles or that bleed or change colour.

TREATMENT

There are numerous traditional remedies for warts, including "selling" them. More practical solutions include dabbing them with fresh sap from dandelions or greater celandine at least three times a day, or applying one drop of neat tea tree oil or thuja tincture directly to the warts night and morning.

dandelion

EYE PROBLEMS

Although old herbals contain eye remedies – many of dubious efficacy – for everything from sore eyelids to blindness, it is best to limit home remedies to treating simple infections and inflammations.

BLEPHARITIS

An inflammation of the eyelid, blepharitis can be caused by bacterial infection or occur as an allergic reaction to cosmetics or face creams. The eyelid becomes red and swollen and there may be white scales on the lashes. In chronic cases the eyelid can become ulcerated with a yellow crust.

EASING THE SYMPTOMS

Internally a decoction (see p.103) of echinacea and burdock root can help combat infection. Use one teaspoon of the mix per cup three times a day. Alternatively, take up to 600 mg of echinacea in capsules three times a day. Externally, bathe the eye with an infusion of fennel or red clover, or smear a little fresh *Aloe vera* gel on the eyelid.

CONJUNCTIVITIS

Also known as pink eye, conjunctivitis is an inflammation of the fine membrane (conjunctiva) that covers the eyeball. The eye is red and watering, and there may be severe pain and a "gritty feeling" on blinking and a milky discharge that sticks the eyelids together. Conjunctivitis can be caused by pollutants, drugs, irritants in the eye or infection.

■ Repeat eyebaths as often as possible (see box opposite).

■ Take 5 ml of echinacea tincture, up to 500 mg of garlic extract or 10 drops of myrrh tincture up to three times daily.

HERBAL EYEBATHS

Simmer 15 g of dried herb in 600 ml of water for about 10 minutes until the volume is reduced by about a third to make a sterile decoction. Strain well through a fine tea strainer or muslin bag to remove particles of herb which might irritate the eye. Cool the mixture to lukewarm and use to fill an eyebath. Place this over the eye, lean back so that the eye is well wetted and blink several times. If both eyes are affected, use a fresh eyebath for the second eye or thoroughly clean the first one with boiling water to avoid cross-contamination.

Alternatively, add two drops of a suitable herbal tincture to an eyebath filled with freshly boiled water which has been allowed to cool. If the mixture stings at all, dilute it further, as individual sensitivity can vary.

HERBS FOR EYEBATHS

Complaint	Suitable herbs
Conjunctivitis and blepharitis	Eyebright, agrimony, fennel seeds, marigold, elderflower, chamomile, marshmallow, rose petal, raspberry leaf.
Hay fever	Eyebright, agrimony, raspberry leaf, marigold, chamomile.
"Arc eye" (caused by exposure to bright light, as in welding) and other painful inflammations	Self-heal, eyebright, marigold, elderflower.
Strained or tired eyes	Eyebright, raspberry leaf, marigold, mullein, chamomile.

STYES

A stye is acute inflammation of a gland at the base of an eyelash, usually caused by bacterial infection.

■ Take up to 600 mg or 5 ml of echinacea powder or tincture to combat infections and improve immunity.

■ Apply a little *Aloe vera* gel or marigold cream directly to the stye.

■ To bring the stye to a head, infuse a chamomile tea bag and use as a poultice, or wrap a little grated carrot in a piece of gauze and apply to the stye for an hour or two.

TIRED EYES

Overwork, reading in a poor light, air pollution or sitting in smoky rooms can all contribute to sore, tired eyes.

■ Soak a cotton wool pad in an infusion of eyebright or raspberry leaves and apply to the closed eyes while relaxing in a darkened room for 20 minutes or so. Alternatively, you can use slices of fresh cucumber or raw potato or infused chamomile or fennel tea bags in the same way, or try any of the eyebaths suggested in the chart above.

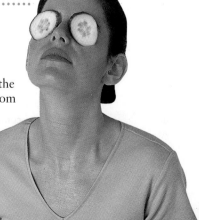

ORAL HEALTH PROBLEMS

R egular dental checks usually keep problems with teeth and gums well under control and any disorders are likely to be minor and self-limiting. However, that doesn't mean they're painless – mouth ulcers or tooth abscesses can cause far more discomfort than their size suggests. Orthodox treatment usually involves antibiotics, but there are plenty of herbal alternatives which can combat infections and inflammations.

TOOTHACHE

Regular dental checks to avoid tooth decay should mean that, aside from obvious damage such as a cracked filling or tooth, the more likely cause of sudden and severe tooth pain will be an abscess or infection. An abscess or infection can often be associated with more general feelings of being unwell or may follow a cold or low-grade flu. Echinacea or garlic tablets will help combat the infection. Persistent toothache with no obvious cause may be associated with sinus problems and catarrh (see p.36).

TREATMENT

For emergency relief of toothache, oil of cloves is one of the most effective remedies. Put a few drops onto a small cotton wool swab and apply to the gum – the oil might sting a little at first, before its anaesthetic properties effectively numb the aching area. You can make a very effective mix for dispersing the abscess from Chinese herbs: mix together equal amounts of Chinese figwort *figwort* root (*xuan shen*) and forsythia *root* berries (*lian xiao*), available from Chinese herb shops, and use them in a decoction (one teaspoon per cup). *forsythia berries* Drink one cup every three or four hours for as long as the pain persists.

GUM PROBLEMS

Bleeding and spongy gums are usually the result of poor oral hygiene and, if untreated, can lead to loss of teeth. Brush the teeth regularly and eat foods that contain roughage and can help clean the teeth as they are chewed. Astringent and antiseptic herbs can be used in mouth washes morning and evening to help bleeding or inflamed gums: use agrimony, bistort, sage, or lady's mantle, or one teaspoon of the tincture of any of *sage* these herbs added to a glass of water.

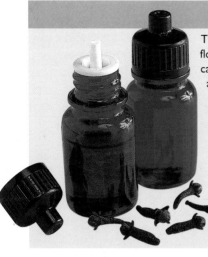

CLOVES

The clove, most familiar as a culinary spice, is the flower bud of an Eastern tree. Cloves are carminative (flatulence-relieving), warming, anodyne (pain-relieving), antiseptic and antispasmodic, and will relieve nausea. The Chinese view them as a good kidney tonic and helpful for the reproductive organs.

Clove oil, produced by steam-distilling the buds, makes a valuable emergency first-aid remedy for toothache and is a popular ingredient for herbal toothpaste. As a warming spice, add cloves to teas for chills and digestive upsets – the flavour can make other herbal brews more palatable.

MOUTH ULCERS

Usually found on the tongue, roof of the mouth, and inside the cheeks, mouth ulcers (aphtha or aphthous stomatitis) start with a red, sore patch of blisters erupting to produce a painful greyish white ulcer. They may occur singly or in groups, and most people suffer from them at some time. The cause is uncertain, though sometimes there is an obvious reason, such as ill-fitting dentures. They are more likely when the sufferer is tired, overstressed or fighting infections, and are often associated with digestive disorders, stomach upsets and yeast infections. They usually clear of their own accord after a week or so.

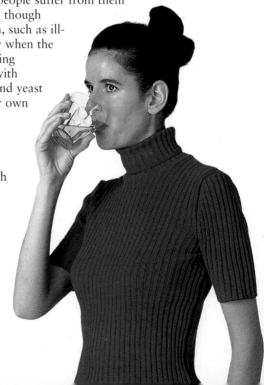

TREATMENT

■ If the problem is recurrent, take ginseng or garlic capsules for a month to boost the immune system.

■ Use herbal mouth washes containing bistort, sage, raspberry leaves, marigold or chamomile infusions. Alternatively, use 10 drops of myrrh tincture added to a glass of warm water.

■ Supplements of evening primrose oil, zinc and yoghurt will help improve general immunity and health.

DIGESTIVE UPSETS

Minor stomach upsets, gastritis and indigestion are usually self-limiting and can generally be solved with simple home remedies. The herbal repertoire is especially rich in digestive remedies, with plants that can stimulate the digestion, reduce acidity, calm over-activity, protect the delicate lining of the digestive tract and help liver function.

INDIGESTION

Indigestion can be caused by rushing meals, tension, wearing tight belts, eating irregularly, or eating too many rich foods. Symptoms can include chest pain, difficulty breathing, wind, nausea and heartburn, or reflux of acid from the stomach into the oesophagus or throat. Recurrent indigestion may indicate a serious underlying disorder, so seek professional help. Indigestion can be confused with heart pain from disorders like angina.

TREATMENT

dill

■ Chamomile and lemon balm help to reduce tension.

■ For mild indigestion, drink a cup of standard infusion of any of the following herbs after meals: fennel seed, cardamom seed, bitter orange, dill seed, ginger, cinnamon, galangal or peppermint.

■ Meadowsweet, Irish moss, dandelion, bogbean, centaury and slippery elm can combat acidity and high acid secretions which could lead to ulcers.

■ Drink a tea containing equal amounts of fennel, bogbean, meadowsweet and lemon balm (two teaspoons of the mix per cup) before a meal.

FOOD POISONING

Symptoms include vomiting, diarrhoea and abdominal pain. The cause is usually an infecting bacteria such as *Salmonella*, *E.coli*, or *Listeria*. Food poisoning can be life-threatening for the elderly, young or ill.

TREATMENT
For emergency treatment before professional help arrives, add a teaspoon of ginger, galangal, cinnamon or cayenne tincture to half a glass of warm water and take one or two sips every few minutes. If you can keep them down, swallow two or three garlic tablets as well. To rehydrate, drink glasses of warm water containing two teaspoons each of salt and sugar.

GASTRITIS

Gastritis is an inflammation of the stomach lining, often caused by overindulgence in rich foods and alcohol, although nervous problems, smoking, stress or vitamin deficiency can also be to blame. Typical symptoms are similar to those of food poisoning, with nausea, vomiting, abdominal pain and diarrhoea, but usually less severe, and other people who have eaten the same meal are unlikely to be affected.

TREATMENT

Herbal remedies include demulcents to protect the stomach lining and the same carminatives used for indigestion. Avoid irritant foods, such as spices, tea, coffee, alcohol, fried foods and pickles. Instead of occasional large meals, eat little and often.

■ Soothing herbal remedies include slippery elm, marshmallow, meadowsweet, liquorice, fenugreek and chamomile.

■ Simmer two teaspoons of fenugreek seeds in a cup of water for 10–15 minutes and then strain this over a teaspoon of dried chamomile and add more boiling water, if needed, to make up the cup.

■ A traditional French remedy is to mix one teaspoon each of lemon balm, fennel seeds and peppermint per cup of infusion and drink as often as required.

HANGOVERS

Remedies to prevent a hangover include slippery elm tablets to coat the stomach and reduce alcohol absorption and an infusion of milk thistle seeds to protect the liver. The symptoms – dry mouth, thirst, irritability and tiredness – call for herbs that soothe the digestion and normalize liver function.

■ Make a tea containing equal amounts of meadowsweet, bogbean, chamomile and agrimony (two teaspoons of the mix per cup), add a pinch of powdered ginger and a teaspoon of honey, and drink as often as necessary. Strong black tea without milk or sugar will soothe the lower bowel if there is diarrhoea.

■ Evening primrose can regulate liver function: take 1 g in capsules in the morning, washed down with a glass of water containing 2 g of soluble vitamin C, and take a second glass of water containing the juice of a lemon to wash the poisons out of the system.

■ Eat plenty of bananas and oranges to restore the body's potassium levels.

NAUSEA AND VOMITING

There are many causes of nausea and vomiting, some of them related to other digestive upsets, such as gastritis, hangovers or indigestion. The sickness may also be caused by conditions ranging from migraine, motion sickness and pregnancy to liver disease or life-threatening fevers. If the cause is uncertain and symptoms persist, seek professional help.

TREATMENT

■ In minor cases, herbal anti-emetics are ideal. Ginger and galangal are among the most effective remedies. Black horehound is also effective, though many people find the smell unpleasant and nauseating in itself.

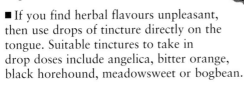

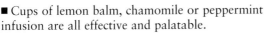
liquorice root

■ If you find herbal flavours unpleasant, then use drops of tincture directly on the tongue. Suitable tinctures to take in drop doses include angelica, bitter orange, black horehound, meadowsweet or bogbean.

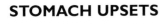

■ Cups of lemon balm, chamomile or peppermint infusion are all effective and palatable.

■ Chew a piece of liquorice root or slippery elm tablets.

STOMACH UPSETS

Gastritis (see previous page), gastro-enteritis – a non-specific term suggesting infection by some invading micro-organism – or some sort of ulceration are the usual causes of stomach upset. However, any acute abdominal pain needs immediate professional attention. Underlying causes can include life-threatening conditions such as pancreatitis, appendicitis or ectopic pregnancy, so do not delay seeking professional treatment.

COLDS AND FLU

Stomach upsets can also be linked to chills and feverish colds or "gastric flu". In such cases, warming herbs such as cayenne, cinnamon, galangal and ginger may be helpful. Simmer a teaspoon of grated fresh galangal or ginger root in a cup of water for 10–15 minutes, strain, and then add a pinch of powdered cayenne or cinnamon before drinking. Repeat as necessary.

STRESS

Stomach discomfort that does not appear to be caused by a specific illness may be stress-related. Many people readily admit to a "nervous tummy" and there is usually some obvious tension or anxiety that has triggered the condition. Lemon balm or chamomile taken in infusion are ideal in such instances, as both these herbs will help to normalize digestive function as well as relaxing the nervous system.

WIND

Gas in the stomach and intestines can be produced by inadequate digestive function as well as by foods such as beans and cabbage. Flatulence can be accompanied by abdominal bloating and cramps and may very occasionally be an indication of some underlying health problem.

PREVENTION

- Avoiding culprit foods or adding carminative herbs and spices when cooking is often sufficient. Caraway, cardamom, cloves, coriander seeds, dill, fennel, garlic, ginger, marjoram, mustard, parsley, sage and thyme are all effective carminatives, and adding them to dishes will reduce any risk of flatulence. Old cookbooks often recommend cooking beans or cabbage with pepper.

- Alternatively, drink a cup of tea made from any of these herbs after each meal – fennel is readily available in tea bags so it is a useful preventative when travelling.

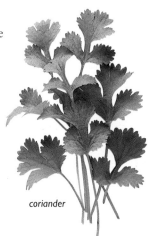

coriander

SLIPPERY ELM

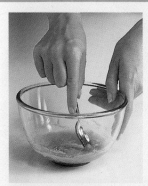

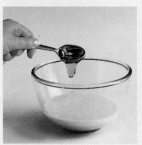

The bark from this North American tree, also known as the red elm, was used by the Native Americans as a remedy for sore throats, digestive problems and wounds, as a poultice for boils, and to ease childbirth. Strips of bark were later used as a mechanical irritant to cause abortion and this use became so widespread that the herb was banned in many countries. Today, only powdered slippery elm bark can be imported into many parts of Europe and sale of bark strips is illegal.

Slippery elm is a highly mucilaginous herb which is soothing, demulcent (soothes irritation) and nutrient and is often use to coat the stomach and provide protection in gastritis, heartburn and ulceration. As a valuable nutrient it makes a useful gruel in convalescence. Mix a teaspoon into a paste with a little water, then stir this into 250 ml of scalded milk and add a teaspoon of honey and a sprinkling of ground cinnamon. Used externally, slippery elm makes an effective drawing ointment for splinters and boils, and can also soothe wounds and burns.

EARS AND NOSE

Both earache and nosebleeds can be symptoms of more serious health problems and in many cases professional treatment is essential. Ear problems, especially in children, can lead to deafness if untreated. Home herbal remedies can be ideal for minor problems but if the symptoms are persistent or severe, see your doctor or medical herbalist.

EARACHE

There are many causes of ear pain – some of them minor and self-limiting, others potential major health hazards. Simple earache will generally resolve within 24 hours but if it persists, seek professional help.

MIDDLE EAR INFECTION

This may start with tonsillitis or a similar infection and spread to the middle ear. There is usually associated fever and there may be a discharge from the ear if the drum bursts. A professional should check whether the ear drum has perforated.

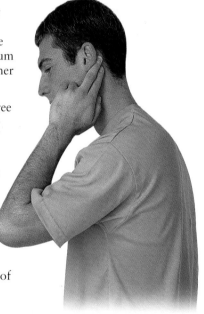

- If the drum is still intact, put two or three drops of warm infused St. John's wort or mullein oil into the ear and cover with a small cotton wool plug.

- Garlic oil is also effective – prick a garlic pearle with a pin and extract the oil.

- Herbal antibiotics, such as garlic and echinacea, will help combat infection.

- Massaging the mastoid bone (behind the ear) with a mixture of 10 drops each of lavender and tea tree oil in a teaspoon of almond oil can also bring relief.

BLOCKED EUSTACHIAN TUBE

Severe ear pain with an unpleasant throbbing sensation can be associated with a blockage in the Eustachian tube (which runs through to the nasal cavity); this can be related to catarrh or sinus problems. Excess catarrh can cause temporary deafness and a blocked sensation in one or both ears.

- Nasal decongestants and steam inhalations can combat catarrh.

- 5 ml of echinacea taken three times a day will fight the infection.

- Drink a cup of infusion containing equal amounts of elder flower, eyebright and mullein (two teaspoons of the mix per cup) as required.

OUTER EAR INFECTION

Itching and irritation in the ear can be caused by local infection in the outer ear; it is common among those who do a lot of swimming or water sports. Fungal infections picked up in the water are often to blame.

■ Bathe the ear frequently with a warm marigold infusion.

■ Use mullein or garlic oil ear drops.

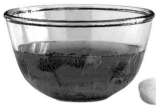

marigold infusion

■ Drink a cup of an infusion containing equal amounts of nettles, cleavers, red clover and marigold (use two teaspoons of the mixture per cup and drink three times a day).

■ Taking echinacea (600 mg capsules or 5 ml tincture three times a day) will also help to combat any infection.

NOSEBLEEDS

Injury, colds and catarrh are the most common causes of nosebleeds. In some cases, the blood vessels in the nose are particularly fragile or near the surface so even minor irritation or blowing too hard can trigger bleeding. Persistent or severe nosebleeds can suggest high blood pressure and can be a problem for the elderly due to weakened blood vessels. If a heavy nosebleed persists for some hours, seek professional help.

■ For minor bleeds, the usual treatment is to simply pinch your nose and bend forward, breathing through your mouth meanwhile. This will usually be effective within a few minutes.

■ A traditional herbal remedy is to insert a yarrow leaf into the affected nostril – the plant's finely divided leaves form a web to encourage clotting while the herb also has styptic qualities (causes blood vessels to contract). Pulped nettle leaves can be used in the same way.

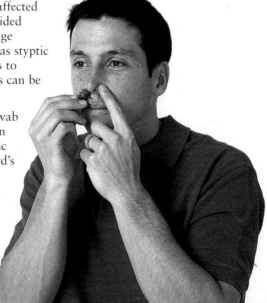

■ Soak a small cotton-wool swab in a tincture or strong infusion made from any suitably styptic herb – yarrow, nettle, shepherd's purse, any of the cranesbill family, marigold, tormentil, oak bark or witch hazel.

■ Drinking a cup of nettle, marigold, shepherd's purse or lady's mantle infusion will also help.

SHOCKS AND SPASMS

Two of the most useful ingredients in the first-aid box for shocks and spasms are Dr Bach's Rescue Remedy and homoeopathic arnica extracts (Arnica 6X). Both are ideal for any nervous upset, accident, traumatic injury or shock and encourage rapid healing.

FAINTING

Any interruption in blood flow to the head will lead to fainting and loss of consciousness. This can be be caused by slowing of the heart beat due to an emotional shock, low blood pressure, blood loss or simply by standing still for too long so that too much blood pools in the legs. Typical early signs of faintness include pallor, sweating and yawning.

TREATMENT

At the first hint of faintness sit or lie down to avoid injury if you fall. Raise your legs above your head, either by bending forward with your head between your knees or lying on the floor with your legs on a chair.

■ Place a drop of Dr Bach's Rescue Remedy on the tongue.

■ A useful standby for those with a tendency to faint is to keep a small bottle of camphor or rosemary oil handy and smell that – it will help to boost the circulation.

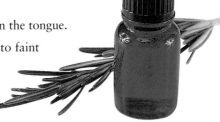

■ Drink a cup of weak chamomile infusion on regaining consciousness to help restore normality.

rosemary oil

CRAMP

This sudden contraction of the muscles is associated with oxygen starvation or low salt levels due to excessive sweating. Rubbing the affected muscles vigorously or stretching can generally bring relief.

■ For mild cases drink a cup of wood betony, St. John's wort, skullcap, lime flower tea, or chamomile singly or in combination (one teaspoon per cup).

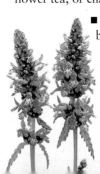

■ For more severe problems, take a cup of decoction of cramp bark and wild yam or 5 ml of the combined tinctures.

■ Massaging with aromatic oils can help – mix 10 drops each of marjoram, pine and lavender oils in 25 ml of almond oil and use on the affected areas as required.

■ For persistent night-time leg cramps, bathe the legs with cramp bark infusion or apply cramp bark cream before going to bed.

wood betony

SHOCK

Emotional upset, sudden fear or physical trauma such as electric shock or a traffic accident can cause shock, in which the blood pressure becomes dangerously lowered. Typical symptoms include a cold sweat, rapid pulse, breathlessness, giddiness and shivering.

- Take warm bed rest and drink plenty of fluids.

- Smelling camphor or rosemary oil can help.

- Drink herbal teas to improve fluid balance and calm the nerves – make an infusion containing equal amounts of sage and skullcap (one teaspoon of each per cup) and drink a mug of slippery elm gruel (see p.27).

- A few drops of Dr Bach's Rescue Remedy directly on the tongue will speed recovery. Rescue Remedy is available as a cream for use where there is loss of consciousness – smear a little on the temples.

rosemary oil

MINOR HEADACHES

There are many causes of headache, including tension, digestive upsets, fevers, sinus problems, nasal congestion, eye-strain, exhaustion, or menstrual irregularities. Finding the cause is important, especially if the headaches are severe or persistent. Seek professional help for any sudden or severe headache that lasts more than 48 hours or is accompanied by vomiting, a stiff neck, slurred speech, double vision, rash or fever. See p.71 for more information on severe headaches and migraine and p.36 for sinus headaches. For minor headaches, herbal remedies make an effective alternative to painkillers.

TREATING MINOR HEADACHES
- Try infusions of any of the following, either singly or in combination (use up to two teaspoons of dried herb in total per cup): St. John's wort, lavender, wood betony, passionflower, rosemary, chamomile, vervain or lime flowers.

- Alternatively, take valerian tablets (500 mg up to three times a day) or massage the temples with 5 drops of lavender, chamomile or rosemary oils in a teaspoon of almond oil.

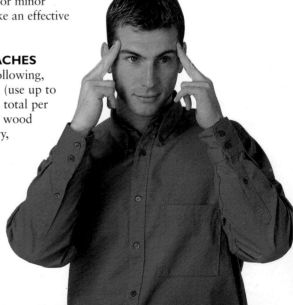

SKIN IRRITATIONS

Skin irritations from insects or allergens are generally minor and self-limiting, but very uncomfortable. Many of the herbs traditionally used for these conditions are available as over-the-counter products, which are well worth keeping in the first-aid box.

SKIN RASHES AND ITCHING

An allergic reaction causing irritant weals on the skin is variously described as urticaria, hives or nettle rash. Urticaria is often caused by food allergies – common culprits include shellfish and strawberries – as well as orthodox drugs like antibiotics. Contact irritants such as cosmetics, perfumes, cleaning materials and a lengthy list of common garden plants including stinging nettles, hops, runner bean tendrils, borage, yarrow and chamomile can also be a problem.The red blotches usually fade within a few hours although in severe cases there may be anaphylactic shock (see Insect Bites and Stings, below).

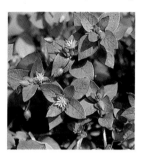

■ Herbal creams will relieve the itching and soreness. Wash the area with an infusion of chickweed (*left*), elder flowers, plantain or chamomile and apply creams containing any of the same herbs.

■ Borage juice is also very soothing – it is available commercially, or you could process a handful of leaves in a food blender and strain the juice.

■ Burdock, marshmallow and nettle leaves can be drunk in infusion for their anti-histamine effect.

INSECT BITES AND STINGS

In rare cases bee or wasp stings can lead to a life-threatening allergic reaction, so emergency medical treatment is vital. Symptoms include dizziness, sickness, breathing problems and marked swelling. If you do not have an allergy, try the following:

■ Bathe the wound with warm water containing one teaspoon of marigold tincture per cup. For a wasp sting, wash with vinegar.

■ Remove a bee sting with a clean needle, then apply a soothing cream containing lemon balm, sage, marigold, *Aloe vera* or St. John's wort.

■ Apply a slice of fresh onion to the area.

■ If a bite becomes infected, use echinacea or tea tree cream, or bathe it frequently with one teaspoon of tea tree oil diluted in one teaspoon of water.

INSECT REPELLENT

To deter mosquitoes and gnats in the summer, make a wash of lemon balm (melissa) or citronella oils in water (20 drops of oil to 25 drops of water). Keep the mixture in a plastic spray bottle and apply liberally to exposed skin.

BURNS AND SUNBURN

Only the most minor burns (less than 5 cm in diameter) should be treated at home – anything larger is a potential medical emergency and professional help should be sought without delay.

For sunburn, prevention is better than cure: stay in the shade if possible, and when in direct sun cover up with light clothing or wear a sun cream with a suitably high protection factor.

TREATMENT

■ Cool a minor burns under cold running water for several minutes to reduce the risk of blistering, or use an ice pack – a bag of frozen peas is ideal.

■ Once the immediate pain has eased, apply either St. John's wort or *Aloe vera* cream to the burn or use the sap from a fresh *Aloe vera* leaf.

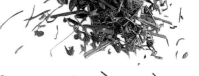

St. John's wort

■ Cover the burn with a loose bandage to prevent accidentally bursting any blisters that form.

■ An alternative treatment is to apply infused St. John's wort oil to minor burns (it is well worth keeping a bottle of the oil in the kitchen for this purpose). Add up to 20 percent lavender oil to make the mixture even more cooling and effective.

■ Sunburn can be treated in much the same way as minor burns: cool the affected area and dab on a soothing oil or cream.

CHILBLAINS

Chilblains are the result of the body's attempts to conserve heat in cold weather, so keep the hands and feet warm to prevent their forming. Habitual sufferers can improve their circulation with stimulating herbs like angelica, cinnamon twigs, prickly ash bark or ginger. Use these in decoctions (one teaspoon per cup) or take up to 20 drops of tincture in water three times daily. Ginkgo will also improve the peripheral blood circulation.

EASING DISCOMFORT

The irritant discomfort of chilblains can be eased by arnica cream (don't use on broken skin), *Aloe vera* gel, marigold cream, or bathing the area with ten drops of myrrh or oak tincture in a cup of warm water.

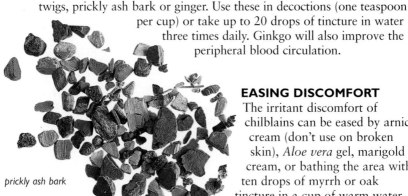

prickly ash bark

CORNS AND CALLUSES

Corns are small, often painful, areas of thickened and hard skin on the toes; calluses are more widespread areas of hard skin on the soles of the feet, fingers or palms. Both are caused by constant friction or pressure, which causes the skin cells to reproduce, thus thickening the skin. The pain of corns is due to pressure on the nerve endings. Once the cause of the friction is removed, corns and calluses will clear of their own accord, although especially painful patches are best treated by a chiropodist.

TREATMENT

■ Thick felt rings placed on the corns can relieve pressure from shoes.

■ Rub corns with crushed garlic cloves or raw onion to draw out any pus.

■ Rubbing the feet with fresh plantain leaves or soaking them in a decoction of oak bark will help to strengthen the skin and can be an effective preventative.

■ Regularly apply an oak lotion or cream on your hands if you are likely to develop calluses from such repeated activities as rowing or playing a musical instrument.

■ To bring relief from painful hard skin, soak your feet in a bowl of hot water containing five drops of lavender oil. Dry the feet, then massage them using a little lavender oil diluted in almond oil (five drops of lavender to a teaspoon of almond oil).

INFUSED ST. JOHN'S WORT OIL

To make your own infused St. John's wort oil, fill a large clear glass jar with the flowering tops of the stems collected during the summer and cover with a good quality vegetable oil, such as cold-pressed safflower or sunflower oil. Leave the jar on a sunny windowsill for two or three weeks; it will gradually turn red as the plant extracts are absorbed. Strain the mixture through a jelly bag or wine press and store in clean dark glass bottles away from direct sunlight. For a stronger mixture repeat the process using this red oil and a fresh supply of St. John's wort flowers.

HERBS FOR THE BODY

This section looks at some of the more serious or chronic health problems. Self-help is appropriate in mild cases or where the diagnosis is certain, but if you are uncertain of the exact condition or if symptoms worsen or do not respond to treatment, seek professional help, either from a doctor or a professional herbal therapist (see p. 8). As well as home-made remedies, a wide range of licensed herbal products of proven efficacy are available.

All the ailments covered here will respond well to herbal treatment. However, the time that treatment takes will vary significantly between ailments. For example, an arthritic problem could take three months to show any improvement on a herbal health regime, while herbs prescribed to lower blood sugar levels could have an immediate effect.

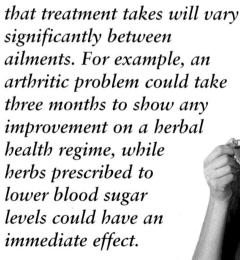

NASAL PROBLEMS

The fine mucous membranes coated in tiny hairs which cover the nasal passages are in the front line, defending our bodies from invading allergens, toxins and infections. The more invading organisms they have to cope with, then the more mucus they produce – as any country-dweller who spends a day being bombarded with city traffic fumes will readily appreciate. Herbs can help to strengthen these vital membranes and repair them when the invaders become overwhelming. Smoking attacks the membranes and increases catarrh – give it up.

2

CATARRH AND SINUSITIS

Catarrh can be associated with the common cold (see pp.16–17) and allergic reactions. It may stay in the upper respiratory tract, causing nasal congestion, or the mucus may run into the lower airways and be coughed up as phlegm. There are different types of catarrh – ranging from the thick yellow variety which is difficult to shift to a watery, semi-permanent drip.

TREATING CATARRH

Many herbalists regard thick catarrh as a "hot" problem to be treated with cooling remedies; suitable herbs include white horehound, wood betony, chamomile or golden rod. Watery catarrh is regarded as "cold" and is more likely to respond to warming herbs such as angelica, hyssop, coltsfoot or eucalyptus. Use the herbs in teas (one teaspoon per cup), steam inhalations or tinctures (20–60 drops per dose).

> **TIP**
>
> Suppressing tears can block the upper respiratory tract and may contribute to sinus problems.

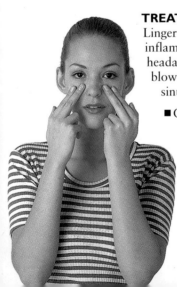

TREATING SINUSITIS

Lingering catarrh can encourage bacteria and cause painful inflammation of the sinuses, often associated with headaches which worsen when bending forward or blowing the nose. To shift the catarrh causing painful sinuses:

■ Gradually stir in drops of bayberry tincture or chamomile or yarrow oil to elder flower cream (often sold as a hand cream) until the cream will not absorb any more. Massage the cream into the area around the cheek bones, bridge of the nose and beneath the eyes.

■ Drink a tea containing equal amounts of elder flowers, yarrow and thyme, and use steam inhalations to which you have added chamomile flowers or a few drops of sandalwood oil.

USING STEAM INHALATION

Pour I litre of boiling water over one tablespoon of dried herb in a mixing bowl, or add five to ten drops of an appropriate essential oil to the hot water. Cover both your head and the bowl with a towel and inhale the steam for as long as you can. Avoid going into a cold atmosphere for 30 minutes after the inhalation. Suitable herbs for allergic problems (such as hay fever and asthma) include chamomile or yarrow flowers. Sandalwood, eucalyptus, pine, thyme or lavender oils or benzoin tincture work well for catarrh and sinus problems.

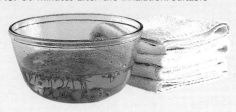

2

HAY FEVER AND ALLERGIC RHINITIS

Hay fever sufferers are sensitive to pollen. The types of pollen which can trigger an attack range from flowering trees in spring to the spores from the autumn mushrooms. Catarrhal problems that are triggered by house dust, animal hairs or car fumes are usually labelled as allergic rhinitis. Both conditions produce similar symptoms associated with the body's production of histamine in response to the irritant. These include sneezing, itchy, sore and watering eyes, a running nose and drowsiness.

PREVENTION AND RELIEF
■ To help strengthen the mucous membranes before an allergic reaction begins, make an infusion by simmering one teaspoon of dandelion root in 500 ml of water and then pouring this over two teaspoons each of dried elder flower, vervain and white horehound. Drink one cup of the infusion three times a day.

■ Ease the symptoms during an attack by taking eyebright capsules (600 mg per dose) once or twice a day as needed.

eyebright capsules

ANTI-CATARRH DIET

■ Try to eliminate mucus-forming foods – such as refined carbohydrates, dairy products and alcohol – completely from your diet for a few days.

■ If you are otherwise fit and well, try a fruit fast for 24 hours to help clear toxic wastes from the body – eat only fruit, up to three or four pieces per meal, and drink only water and fruit juices.

■ Take zinc and vitamin C supplements to help strengthen your immune system generally and combat infection.

CHEST PROBLEMS

There are plenty of herbal cough remedies for treating respiratory disorders – strong expectorants to encourage the production of phlegm; cough suppressants, which can ease a persistent dry, tickling cough; demulcents which will soothe irritated mucous membranes; and anti-bacterials to combat infection.

COUGHS

Coughing is the body's natural reaction to any blockage in the airways – from dust to excess mucus following an infection. Persistent coughing can be a symptom of serious illness so seek professional help for any cough which does not improve with simple treatments or where there is no obvious cause. See a doctor if you cough up blood or blood-streaked phlegm. Use herbs singly or in combinations in teas, syrups or tinctures. Garlic, thyme and hyssop are antibacterial and can be used in cough remedies.

PRODUCTIVE COUGHS

Stimulating herbal expectorants should be used for congestive conditions to encourage productive coughing and clear phlegm. They include: balm of Gilead, blood root, mouse ear, white horehound, cowslip, sweet violets and elecampane. A typical mix for a productive cough with infected phlegm might be thyme, white horehound and elecampane.

DRY COUGHS

Demulcents (marshmallow, plantain, mullein and Irish moss) soothe irritated mucous membranes. Relaxing expectorants (coltsfoot, hyssop, marshmallow, plantain, liquorice, aniseed and pleurisy root) have a soothing effect and loosen phlegm. Suppressants such as wild cherry, aniseed or wild lettuce can treat a lingering or nervous cough. For a dry irritating cough try a mixture of liquorice, hyssop and marshmallow.

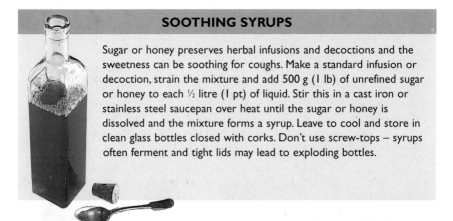

SOOTHING SYRUPS

Sugar or honey preserves herbal infusions and decoctions and the sweetness can be soothing for coughs. Make a standard infusion or decoction, strain the mixture and add 500 g (1 lb) of unrefined sugar or honey to each ½ litre (1 pt) of liquid. Stir this in a cast iron or stainless steel saucepan over heat until the sugar or honey is dissolved and the mixture forms a syrup. Leave to cool and store in clean glass bottles closed with corks. Don't use screw-tops – syrups often ferment and tight lids may lead to exploding bottles.

ASTHMA

Asthma occurs when the small bronchial tubes in the lungs tighten and fill with sticky mucus, making it difficult for the sufferer to breathe out and resulting in a characteristic wheeze. It can be life-threatening and needs professional medical treatment, so don't rely on self-help remedies.

AVOIDING ATTACKS

■ Sufferers should identify and avoid things that are likely to trigger an attack – asthma may be associated with a food allergy, stress or traffic fumes.

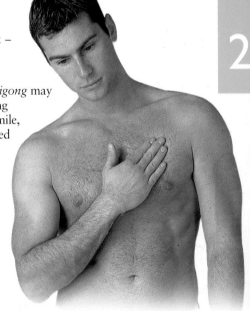

■ Relaxation techniques such as yoga or *qigong* may help combat stress, as will drinking calming herbal infusions, such as skullcap, chamomile, or wood betony, in preference to caffeinated drinks such as tea, coffee and cola.

■ Minor attacks may be averted by steam inhalations using a mixture of thyme leaves and chamomile flowers. Alternatively, massage the chest with a mixture of five drops each of eucalyptus, peppermint, thyme and aniseed oil in two teaspoons of almond or infused comfrey oil.

■ To strengthen the lungs, drink regular cups of coltsfoot, white horehound, mullein, hyssop, elecampane or plantain tea, or take Korean ginseng (600 mg daily).

BRONCHITIS

Bronchitis is an inflammation of the airways. It is a serious condition which is aggravated by cold and damp and is a major cause of early death. It generally needs professional medical treatment.

EASING SYMPTOMS

■ Apply a chest rub made from five drops each of pine, thyme, eucalyptus and angelica oils in two teaspoons of almond oil.

■ For acute episodes drink a tea made by combining a decoction, containing equal amounts of elecampane root and wild cherry bark, with an infusion containing equal amounts of marshmallow leaf and thyme.

■ For chronic bronchitis, drink a decoction of equal amounts of elecampane, pleurisy root and cowslip with two teaspoons of horsetail juice added to each dose two or three times a day. Thyme tea will help clear mucus.

THROAT PROBLEMS

Sore throats are among the most common ailments. Although throat problems are generally minor and self-limiting they can occasionally be more serious, as with croup in young children or peritonsillar abscesses (quinsy). If symptoms persist or there is an accompanying fever, seek professional help.

2

SORE THROAT

A sore throat is a symptom of many disorders and may be the first sign of an infection such as flu, laryngitis or German measles. Recurrent sore throats – often due to *Streptococcus* infection – are common in young adults and are usually linked to exhaustion, overwork and stress.

REMEDIES
■ Take 5 ml tincture of echinacea or 600 mg in echinacea capsules three times a day to combat the infection.

■ Drink plenty of fresh lemon juice mixed with warm water, adding a spoonful of honey to each glass.

■ Drink cups of infusion made from equal amounts of golden rod, marshmallow leaves and sage (use one to two teaspoons of the mix per cup).

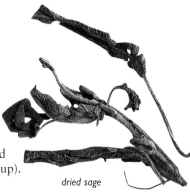
dried sage

HERBAL AND FRUIT GARGLES

Regularly gargling with one of these remedies (every 30–60 minutes during the day) will hasten recovery from a sore throat.

■ Add 5ml of echinacea tincture to half a glass of warm water and use it to gargle with before swallowing.

■ Pour a cup of boiling water onto one teaspoon of red sage, thyme, lady's mantle, rosemary or raspberry leaf (or a mixture of them). Allow to cool, then strain.

■ Dilute half a glass of pineapple juice with an equal amount of water and add the fresh juice of a lemon. The same mixture can be used to spray the back of the throat during the day.

TONSILLITIS

The tonsils are small areas of lymphatic tissue at the back of the throat which help to protect the body from infection – when they become inflamed or infected the result is tonsillitis. Tonsillitis can be severe and requires professional medical help. Symptoms include a sore throat, problems swallowing, fever and obvious spots or a white discharge around the tonsils. In severe cases the tonsil can become filled with pus, causing an abscess or quinsy which can need surgical treatment.

Recurrent inflammation can often indicate some underlying stress, such as a food allergy or overwork.

TREATMENT

■ Take echinacea (5 ml of tincture three times daily) or garlic (up to 1 g in capsules daily) to combat infection.

■ Gargle or spray the back of the throat with a mixture of pineapple and lemon juice (see box, left).

■ A cold compress around the neck made by soaking a cloth in distilled witch hazel can also help ease the discomfort.

distilled witch hazel

LARYNGITIS

Laryngitis is an inflammation of the voice box (larynx) and vocal cords, usually caused by infection. Symptoms include hoarseness or loss of voice, sore throat and fever. Laryngitis is usually self-limiting and minor and can be relieved by talking as little as possible and gargling frequently. Seek professional advice if symptoms persist. The early stages of croup, which always requires professional treatment, can be confused with laryngitis but are usually accompanied by high fever and characteristic cough.

RELIEF FROM LARYNGITIS

A palatable remedy is to sprinkle a teaspoon of powdered cinnamon on one scoop of vanilla ice cream or add two drops of cinnamon oil to a teaspoon of honey and eat three or four times a day. Steam inhalations using five drops of eucalyptus, lavender or sandalwood oil in a basin of boiling water will help. Gargling with an infusion of red sage, raspberry leaf or rosemary (see box, left) should also provide relief.

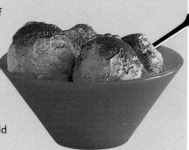

INFECTIONS

2

Recurrent infection can be linked to reduced resistance and an immune system damaged by such factors as stress and food allergies. Tonic herbs as well as many aromatic oils, garlic and echinacea can support the immune system. Echinacea is best for short-term use (up to a week) to combat infections, while tonic herbs should be part of a longer-term strengthening strategy. Korean ginseng can be taken for four weeks at a time or use shiitake mushrooms in soups and stews.

CANDIDIASIS

Yeast infections can cause a wide range of symptoms including digestive upsets, vaginal thrush (see p.83) and aches and pains. Some argue that by-products from the yeast may lead to menstrual irregularities and nervous disorders. *Candida albicans* is the most common of some 60–70 yeasts which can affect the body. They usually cause few problems, but if resistance is weakened by overwork, stress or illness, they proliferate.

PREVENTION AND TREATMENT

■ Avoid foods which encourage yeast proliferation – sugars, alcohol, highly processed foods, refined carbohydrates and dairy products.

pau d'arco

■ Drink three to four cups of marigold infusion daily and use plenty of garlic in cooking.

■ Anti-fungal herbs and immune stimulants such as garlic, echinacea, marigold, myrrh, thuja and *Aloe vera* can be effective. Myrrh and thuja are best taken in tinctures up to ten drops in water per dose. The South American plant pau d'arco is widely available in over-the-counter products recommended for candidiasis.

A NATURAL ANTISEPTIC

Garlic has been used in medicine for at least 5,000 years largely as an antiseptic effective against bacteria and fungi. It is ideal for fighting infection and digestive upsets. It reduces blood cholesterol levels, helping to reduce the risk of heart problems. In the East, garlic is used in low doses for the elderly to improve weak digestive function. Either crush the fresh cloves in milk, use in cooking or take up to 2 g daily in capsules or pearles. Avoid deodorized tablets – the most active components of garlic are the smelliest.

SHINGLES

Shingles is caused by the *Herpes zoster* virus and often involves reactivation of dormant chicken pox virus in adults who have already suffered from the disease in childhood. Shingles is most common in people over 50; in younger people the virus is most likely to be reactivated when the immune system is run down. The first symptoms of shingles are usually a fever, and this is followed by a red, blistering rash along the route of a nerve (such as across the face or chest) and localized pain.

The disease usually eases within three weeks but pain along the affected nerve can persist for months. The severity of the attack often depends on the nerve involved – shingles affecting eyes or mouth can be especially unpleasant and professional treatment should be sought.

2

TREATMENT

■ To combat the virus, take echinacea (5 ml of tincture or 600 mg in capsules) three or four times a day.

■ Drink cups of tea made from an infusion of equal amounts of passionflower, St. John's wort and nettles (use two teaspoons of the infusion per cup).

■ Relieve the rash with *Aloe vera* sap, ice packs, a tea tree oil wash (one teaspoon of oil mixed into a cup of water) or slippery elm paste. Vervain or St. John's wort creams may also help.

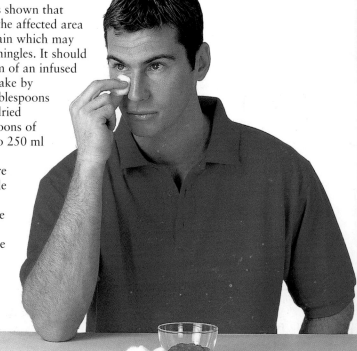

■ Recent research has shown that applying cayenne to the affected area can ease the severe pain which may follow an attack of shingles. It should be applied in the form of an infused oil, which you can make by adding one to two tablespoons of chopped fresh or dried chillies (or two teaspoons of powdered cayenne) to 250 ml of sunflower oil and simmering the mixture over water in a double saucepan for two to three hours. Strain the oil through a fine muslin cloth and leave to cool before use.

GLANDULAR FEVER

Glandular fever (infectious mononucleosis) is most common among teenagers and young adults. The disease has a long incubation period and can commonly affect school friends over several months. It is thought to be caused by the Epstein-Barr virus and the usual symptoms include enlarged and tender lymph nodes in the neck, armpits and groin with loss of appetite, headache, fever, sore throat and general lethargy.

2

While the actual symptoms may persist for several weeks, sufferers are also left feeling drained and debilitated for months. Sometimes apparent recovery is followed by relapse – especially if the patient is working hard or under stress. Often school leavers

cleavers

who have suffered with glandular fever find that recurrent bouts of lethargy will coincide with their first year college exams or stresses associated with starting a new job. Always consult your health-care professional in cases of glandular fever and use herbal remedies to support any prescribed treatment.

PROMOTING HEALTH

Herbal treatment combines anti-viral herbs with stimulants to improve digestion and metabolism and to boost energy levels.

■ While the glands are swollen and the disease is at the acute stage, take garlic capsules or echinacea (600 mg capsules or 5 ml of tincture) three times a day to combat the virus. Process enough fresh cleavers in a food-mixer to make two tablespoons of juice when strained, and combine this with a pinch of powdered cayenne and the juice of half a lemon. Repeat this every three to four hours.

■ During the recovery phase, make a tonic decoction by combining equal amounts of elecampane, rosemary leaves and barberry bark. Use one teaspoon per cup for a daily brew, and take 600 mg of Korean ginseng for up to one month after the lymphatic swellings subside.

SKIN PROBLEMS

Our skin is a barometer for our health – glowing with vitality when we feel well, pale and papery when we run out of energy, yellowish in liver disease, dark tinged in food allergy. Our skin is home to millions of assorted micro-organisms which can sometimes cause problems.

ECZEMA

Eczema can vary from the dry, itchy variety with scaly patches to a "weeping" condition with spots resembling small blisters which ooze clear fluid and form a crust. It is often associated with allergies – such as sensitivity to metals in jewellery or clothing, or some sort of masked food allergy – and may be related to stress. Identifying and avoiding the allergic trigger is important.

2

TREATMENT

Herbal treatment is usually based on blood cleansing remedies to clear toxins and reduce any inflammation.

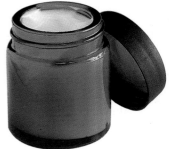

aloe vera cream

■ Drink regular infusions containing equal amounts of figwort, red clover and cleavers. For dry eczema add marigold to the mix (two teaspoons of the herb mixture in total per cup). Alternatively, make a decoction of burdock, dandelion and yellow dock roots and drink a cup three times a day.

■ Marigold or *Aloe vera* creams can be used externally for dry, scaly eczema, while lemon balm cream can help with weeping eczema. Chickweed cream will help to relieve itching.

■ Poor circulation can be a factor, especially in the elderly – add a pinch of powdered cinnamon or ginger to teas or use a combination of melilot and marigold cream if there is varicose eczema (usually dark in colour, associated with varicose veins and affecting the lower leg).

PSORIASIS

Psoriasis is characterized by itchy, dry skin covered with silvery scales that flake off to reveal inflamed, red areas. The knees, legs, elbows, forearm and scalp are commonly affected. Anxiety and stress can exacerbate the problem.

GETTING RELIEF

For minor outbreaks, cleavers cream used externally can be very effective. Also, drink a infusion containing equal amounts of red clover, figwort, skullcap and burdock leaves. Taking devil's claw tablets can help if there is associated arthritis.

devil's claw capsules

CIRCULATORY PROBLEMS

Western medicine often equates the heart with a mechanical pump and regards the blood circulation as the body's plumbing. In Chinese medicine and the Ayurvedic tradition, the heart is far more closely aligned with emotions and spiritual qualities. Some complementary practitioners argue that the high incidence of heart disease in our society is linked not so much to poor diet and lack of exercise but to our spiritual vacuum.

2

IRON-DEFICIENT ANAEMIA

The body uses haemoglobin, a constituent of blood which contains iron, to transport oxygen to the tissues. If the body fails to manufacture enough haemoglobin, we become starved of oxygen. The resulting symptoms include fatigue, breathlessness, pallor, insomnia, dizziness, assorted aches and pains, confusion and reduced resistance to infection.

There are many reasons why a shortfall in haemoglobin might occur. Among the most common are blood loss and a lack of iron through dietary deficiency. Other causes can be life-threatening, as in leukaemia, so professional diagnosis is essential.

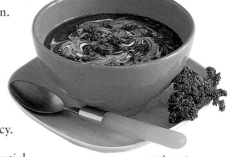
nettle soup

NOURISHING THE BLOOD

■ Efficient iron absorption depends on having enough folic acid and vitamin C, so as well as eating iron-rich foods – such as meat, watercress, apricots and blackcurrants – eat plenty of fruit, whole grains and green vegetables. Parsley and nettles contain vitamin C and iron, so use plenty of parsley to garnish your dishes, or make nettle soup.

■ Bitter herbs will also stimulate digestion and improve absorption of essential nutrients; take two to three drops of gentian or wormwood tincture in a teaspoon of water before meals.

Vegan diets

Vegans can be at risk from anaemia associated with vitamin B$_{12}$ deficiency (known as pernicious anaemia). Professional treatment is essential.

■ In traditional Chinese medicine, Chinese angelica – known as *dang gui* or *tang kwai* – is believed to "nourish the blood" and is often used to treat anaemia. Use pieces of the dried root to flavour soups and stews or take 600 mg daily – it is now available from health food shops in tablet form.

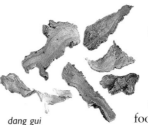
dang gui

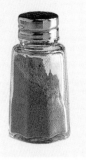

POOR CIRCULATION

Poor circulation can have a range of causes, from heart and circulatory disorders to an inherited tendency for "dead" fingers on cold days. Smokers are particularly at risk from Buerger's disease, a condition which also involves leg pain when walking and which needs professional treatment. A sluggish circulation is often associated with general debility.

TREATMENT

■ For minor circulatory problems or where there is no pathological cause, drink decoctions of warming, circulatory stimulants such as ginger, galangal, cinnamon or prickly ash bark (half to one teaspoon of herb per cup). Rosemary, yarrow and lime flowers also help – mix equal amounts for an infusion and add a clove to each cup.

■ Taking buckwheat or ginkgo tablets as a regular supplement will improve general circulation.

2

ATHEROSCLEROSIS

Hardening of the arteries and the build up of fatty deposits on the walls of blood vessels can result from high cholesterol. It can be associated with blood clots, circulatory disorders and heart disease. Symptoms include poor circulation, headaches, giddiness, pain on exertion or breathlessness.

PREVENTION AND RELIEF

■ Drink a daily cup of infusion containing equal amounts of marigold, lime flowers and hawthorn as a preventative.

■ Garlic is one of the most effective herbs for lowering cholesterol levels.

■ Adding a tablespoon of oat bran to breakfast cereals also helps to reduce cholesterol levels.

■ Buckwheat and ginkgo strengthen the blood vessels. Both can be taken as tablets, while buckwheat can be taken as an infusion up to three times a day.

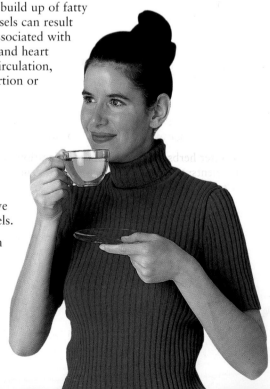

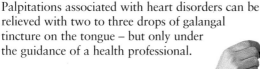

TIP

If nervous tension contributes to high blood pressure, take 5 ml of cramp bark tincture in water three times daily or use commercial valerian tablets.

BLOOD PRESSURE

If you have problems with your blood pressure, seek professional help and use self-help remedies only in mild cases. Do not replace long-term medication with herbs without consulting your doctor.

HIGH BLOOD PRESSURE

High blood pressure is often associated with an increase in the thickness of the blood, atherosclerosis or kidney disorders, although in 90 percent of cases there is no obvious cause. Symptoms include headaches, nose bleeds, dizziness and heart pains. For high blood pressure mix equal amounts of hawthorn, yarrow, motherwort and lime flowers. Take two teaspoons in a cup of hot water up to three times daily.

LOW BLOOD PRESSURE

Low blood pressure can be linked to blood loss, general debility or shock and symptoms can include dizziness, headaches, fainting, anxiety and panic attacks. For low blood pressure mix equal amounts of hawthorn, betony, peppermint and rosemary with a pinch of cayenne powder and take two teaspoons in a cup of hot water up to three times per day.

PALPITATIONS

An awareness of one's heart beating quickly at rest may be caused by anxiety, too much coffee, or a chronic thyroid or heart conditions, so seek professional help. Palpitations associated with heart disorders can be relieved with two to three drops of galangal tincture on the tongue – but only under the guidance of a health professional.

INSTANT REMEDIES

■ Palpitations due to anxiety can be helped by taking ten drops of valerian tincture in a little water every two hours or by drinking an infusion containing equal amounts of motherwort, passionflower and vervain (two teaspoons of the mix per cup) up to three times a day.

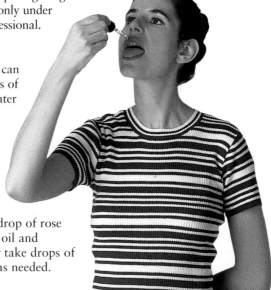

■ For a panic attack, add a drop of rose oil to a teaspoon of almond oil and massage into the temples, or take drops of rose tincture on the tongue as needed.

VARICOSE VEINS

Veins are muscular structures which help to pump blood back to the heart. If the muscles are weakened, for example by obesity, high blood pressure or lack of exercise, the veins in the legs become distended, lengthened and tortuous. Other symptoms include aching legs and hot tingling sensations at night – sometimes described as "formication", or a sensation that ants are crawling across the limbs.

TREATMENT

■ A simple remedy is to raise the end of the bed to help the blood flow back to the heart, and spray the legs each morning for one to two minutes with alternate hot and cold water showers, several times each.

2

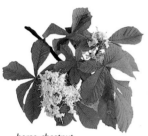

■ Distilled witch hazel or dilute horse chestnut tincture (two teaspoons to 100 ml of water) can be used to bathe the veins. Alternatively, apply horse chestnut or comfrey ointments, but do not massage the veins – dab on lotions or creams as gently as you can.

■ Drink a tea made from equal amounts of motherwort and yarrow (use one teaspoon per cup) with a pinch of cayenne powder added to each cup.

horse chestnut

PILES

Piles, or haemorrhoids, are varicose veins occurring around the rectum. They look and feel like tiny bunches of grapes. Symptoms include pain, anal itching, bleeding and mucous discharge. Piles are the most likely explanation for seeing blood in the lavatory pan after passing stools.

PREVENTION AND RELIEF

■ Taking psyllium seeds once a day as a bulking laxative will help to lubricate the bowel and prevent straining, which causes piles.

■ Apply pilewort ointment (the classic herbal remedy), fresh *Aloe vera* sap or distilled witch hazel frequently during the day. Also drink a tea containing equal amounts of dried pilewort leaves, yarrow, mullein (use two teaspoons of the mix per cup and drink three times daily).

HAWTHORN

Hawthorn is now regarded as an important cardiac tonic which will also improve peripheral circulation, regulate heart rate, normalize blood pressure and improve coronary blood flow. Its use for heart disorders should be in consultation with a medical professional.
It is also an astringent so it can be used in gargles for sore throats or added to teas for diarrhoea.

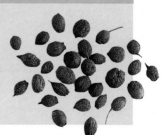

GLANDULAR PROBLEMS

The endocrine glands produce essential hormones. They include the pituitary, thyroid, and adrenal glands, ovaries, testes and parts of the pancreas. Dysfunction can lead to diabetes and thyrotoxicosis and may contribute to many reproductive disorders (see Section 4).Thyroid problems should always be referred to a health-care professional.

2

THYROID

The thyroid gland, located in the throat, produces the hormones that are essential for normal metabolism and mental and physical development.

An excess of thyroid hormones leads to thyrotoxicosis and the body goes into over-drive – the metabolism speeds up leading to weight loss, diarrhoea and sweating. Sufferers are hyperactive.

OVER-ACTIVE THYROID
■ Bugleweed is the specific herb for an over-active thyroid. Make an infusion containing equal amounts of bugleweed and motherwort (two teaspoons per cup, three times a day).

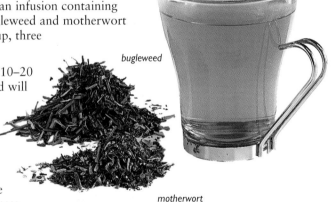

bugleweed

■ Valerian tincture in 10–20 drop doses as required will also help to calm the over-activity. However, take care because this herb can cause hyperactivity in some people and large doses can cause giddiness.

motherwort

UNDER-ACTIVE THYROID
Lack of thyroid hormones leads to cretinism in children and myxoedema in adults. The metabolism is sluggish with constipation, weight gain, apathy and general lethargy. Sufferers have little energy and may appear mentally dull.

■ Bladderwrack is the usual choice for an under-active gland. Like all seaweeds, it is a good source of iodine which is essential to thyroid function. Take commercially available bladderwrack or kelp tablets and drink a tea containing equal amounts of damiana and rosemary to stimulate the system (two teaspoons per cup) three times a day.

■ Avoid eating too much cabbage, cauliflower, spinach, Brussels sprouts, turnip, beans or soya products. Iodine-rich foods can help to ease the condition – try including shellfish and seaweed in your diet.

LATE-ONSET DIABETES

Diabetes in childhood or in young adults usually needs regular insulin injections and professional monitoring. However, late-onset diabetes which usually begins after the age of 60, can often be controlled by diet and simple herbal teas.

TREATMENT

Careful monitoring is essential for this condition and it is best to consult a qualified herbalist before undertaking any treatment. Insulin-dependent diabetics should avoid taking hypoglycaemic herbs, unless they are under professional guidance.

■ Hypoglycaemic herbs lower blood sugar levels. Suitable hypoglycaemic herbs include bladderwrack, goat's rue, stinging nettles, fenugreek seeds, bilberry leaves, *Aloe vera* and garlic.

■ Try a tea made by infusing bilberry and nettle leaves, or simmer a teaspoon of fenugreek seeds in a cup of water for ten minutes. Commercial *Aloe vera* tonics can be useful.

■ Eat plenty of complex carbohydrates (such as brown rice, beans and vegetables) and eat regular portions of banana, papaya, cabbage, lettuce, turnip and olives which encourage the body's insulin production. Try to include plenty of onions and garlic in cooking, or if you do not like the flavour, take garlic supplements.

MAKING INFUSIONS

The leaves, flowers and stems of herbs can easily be made into teas or tisanes by infusing them in water. The usual approach is to add 25 g (1 oz) of dried herb or 75 g (3 oz) of fresh herbs to ½ litre (1 pt) of water that has just gone off the boil (this prevents the herb's oils from dispersing during evaporation). Leave to stand for ten minutes, then strain and drink three wine glasses or cups of the infusion during the day. Store in a covered jug or teapot in a cool place and use within 24 hours. Alternatively, use one to two teaspoons of herb per cup and make a dose at a time.

DIGESTIVE PROBLEMS

Asluggish digestive system can lead to damaging toxins building up in the bowel while over-activity rushes essential nutrients through the system too quickly for effective absorption. A medieval saying was "death dwells in the bowels" suggesting that serious health problems were generally associated with digestive disorders. There are plenty of herbal remedies to choose from to treat the digestive system.

2

CONSTIPATION

This common condition may be just an occasional nuisance, or a symptom of a more serious underlying disorder.

OCCASIONAL PROBLEMS
Occasional constipation is likely to be due to poor diet, stress or lack of exercise.

■ Try a mild bulking laxative such as ispaghula.

■ Mix five drops each of marjoram and rosemary oil in two teaspoons of almond oil and gently massage the tummy and lower abdomen for five minutes each morning.

STRESS-RELATED CONSTIPATION
Constipation that seems to worsen at times of stress may be associated with irritable bowel syndrome (see right).

■ Relaxants can help. Try chamomile tea or a decoction of cramp bark and wild yam (half a teaspoon of each per cup) up to three times a day.

CHRONIC CONDITIONS
Chronic constipation generally has an underlying cause such as anaemia.

■ Strong herbal laxatives are useful in the short-term. Many are available in over-the-counter preparations, including senna, cascara sagrada, alder buckthorn, rhubarb root and aloes.

Griping pains
To combat any griping pains caused by using stronger laxatives, add a carminative such as fennel seeds, ginger, caraway, or lemon balm.

■ A gentler home remedy is a decoction containing equal parts of yellow dock, dandelion root and fennel seeds (two teaspoons of the mix per cup, each morning).

In the elderly, constipation may indicate general weakness. The Chinese treat constipation in the elderly with cannabis seeds and Chinese angelica root (*dang gui*). Try a decoction containing equal amounts of *dang gui* and dandelion root three times a day as well as abdominal massage.

ISPAGHULA OR PSYLLIUM SEEDS

The seeds and husks of two related species – *Plantago ovato* (ispaghula) or *P. psyllium* (psyllium) – are widely used as a bulking laxative for constipation and to ease the symptoms of irritable bowel syndrome.

The seeds swell when moistened to form a glutinous mass which encourages peristalsis and lubricates the bowel. Put a teaspoon of seeds into a cup and fill with boiling water. Once it is cool stir well then drink, seeds and all. Flavouring with fruit juice or mixing the seeds with breakfast cereal can make the remedy more palatable. If taking dry or powdered seeds, drink plenty of water as the seeds will swell and the water is needed to prevent over absorption of gut fluids.

2

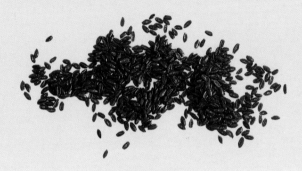

IRRITABLE BOWEL SYNDROME

A range of symptoms can indicate IBS, such as bloating, flatulence, abdominal pain, bouts of diarrhoea and constipation and stools containing mucus and blood or resembling rabbit droppings.

IBS is often associated with food intolerance, the menstrual cycle or stress.

TREATMENT

■ To relieve discomfort and strengthen the digestion, try an infusion made from of agrimony, chamomile and marshmallow leaves (use half a teaspoon of each per cup), with a pinch of caraway seeds or one drop of peppermint emulsion added to each cup. Regular cups of fenugreek-seed tea with a pinch of powdered cinnamon can also help.

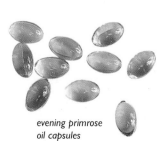

■ If diarrhoea is one of the symptoms, make a decoction of bistort and cramp bark, and add a pinch of powdered cinnamon or a small cinnamon stick to the brew.

■ Try over-the-counter peppermint oil capsules.

■ Women may find that symptoms worsen during menstruation – evening primrose oil (up to 3 g daily) can help.

evening primrose oil capsules

DIARRHOEA

Food poisoning (see p.24) or gastritis resulting from overindulgence (see p.25) can bring on a sudden attack of diarrhoea. Chronic diarrhoea is more likely to be a symptom of some underlying disorder such as Crohn's disease, ulcerative colitis or diverticulosis – all of which require professional treatment.

REMEDIES

■ Strong, cold Indian tea is rich in tannins and will help to astringe and heal a sore gut – drink up to three cups a day.

■ Alternatively, drink an infusion containing equal amounts of raspberry leaves, agrimony and plantain (two teaspoons of the mix per cup) as required.

■ A bout of diarrhoea is dehydrating so it is vital to increase fluid intake, especially for babies and small children; give a glass of water containing one teaspoon of salt and two teaspoons of sugar every few hours.

■ If the diarrhoea is stress related (as is often the case with ulcerative colitis), then drink plenty of calming herbal teas (see pp.108–109).

LIVER AND GALL BLADDER PROBLEMS

Serious liver and gall bladder problems need professional treatment, although herbs can help support other remedies.

LIVER

The liver converts food into vital enzymes, vitamins and clotting agents and stores surplus iron and sugars. It also stops toxins entering the blood.

■ Most of us could do with regular *burdock* cups of cleansing liver remedies. Give your liver an occasional treat with a dandelion and burdock infusion.

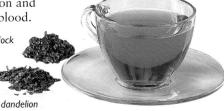

dandelion

GALL BLADDER

The gall bladder stores and concentrates bile produced in the liver. Problems, such as gallstones, may be symptom-free for years, although, developing gall bladder problems are often characterized by discomfort when eating fatty meals, with heartburn and abdominal pain. Symptoms, such as severe abdominal pain,

agrimony shallow breathing, sweating and tenderness in the upper-right abdomen, indicate sudden inflammation.

■ Bitter herbs stimulate the digestion and liquefy bile. Drink an infusion of milk thistle seeds, agrimony and *wormwood* wormwood (one teaspoon of the mix per cup) or try a decoction of equal amounts of fringe tree bark, dandelion root and milk thistle seeds.

milk thistle seeds

OLIVE OIL AND LEMON JUICE REMEDY FOR GALLSTONES

After breakfast eat nothing more until early evening and then drink 30–50 ml of olive oil followed by the fresh juice of one or two lemons diluted with as little warm water as possible. Continue alternating this combination every 20–30 minutes through the evening until you have consumed 500 ml of olive oil and the juice of about nine to ten lemons.

The remnants of the gall stones should then be passed with stools over the next three days appearing as small stones and gritty sand.

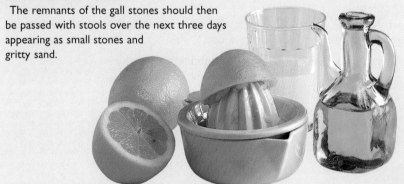

WEAK DIGESTION AND POOR APPETITE

Poor appetite in younger people may indicate an eating disorder which requires professional help. Other causes of appetite loss may include kidney, liver or heart disease, pernicious anaemia, anxiety or stress, or infections.

Poor digestive function and a general lack of interest in food can be a problem as we get older and the food seems to "sit heavily" on the stomach. Elderly people tend to opt for smaller and smaller meals in an attempt to avoid discomfort and bloating.

STIMULATING THE APPETITE

■ Garlic can be an effective appetite stimulant – take a low dose garlic pearle or capsule or simply add half a clove of garlic to dishes and salad dressings.

■ Hawthorn berries are also a popular Chinese remedy for a feeling of fullness – use one teaspoon per cup per day as a decoction.

■ To stimulate digestive function and improve the appetite try drinking fenugreek-seed tea or make an infusion of agrimony, lemon balm and chamomile with a pinch of centaury, and take as needed.

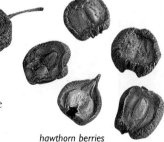

■ A few drops of gentian or wormwood tincture on the tongue before meals will also perk up the appetite.

hawthorn berries

BONES AND MUSCLES

While strains and sprains belong in the first-aid category, herbal remedies are just as effective for long-term chronic ills such as arthritis and fibrositis. Orthodox medicine often depends on powerful painkillers and anti-inflammatories to deal with chronic problems such as fibrositis and arthritis, starting with aspirin and moving to steroid treatment in severe cases. Herbal remedies focus more on clearing toxins from the system while stimulating circulation and metabolism.

2

ARTHRITIS

There are many causes of painful inflammation of the joints, from auto-immune disease and infections to food intolerance or simple wear and tear. Different sorts of arthritis require different treatment, so consult a professional for accurate diagnosis. All types of arthritis improve in warm climates.

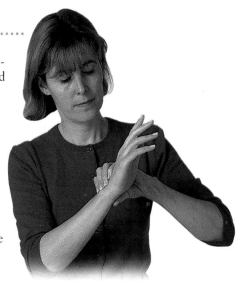

RELIEVING DISCOMFORT
■ Passive exercise – where the joints are manipulated putting no strain on any muscles or ligaments can improve mobility.

■ Cut out all refined carbohydrates, citrus fruits, tomatoes and excessive amounts of red meat.

OSTEOARTHRITIS

Many older people are affected by osteoarthritis, perhaps due to earlier injuries, obesity putting excess demands on weight-bearing joints or wear and tear. The cartilage between the bones of a joint wears away so the bones rub painfully and become deformed.

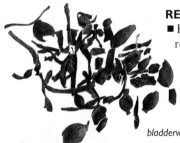

REMEDIES
■ Rubbing infused comfrey oil containing a little rosemary oil into the joints several times a day can ease the pain and repair joint damage.

■ Bladderwrack capsules, tablets or powder used regularly may prevent the progress of the disease.

bladderwrack

RHEUMATOID ARTHRITIS

This serious systemic disorder is potentially crippling and affects most of the joints. It needs professional treatment, although home herbal remedies can be supportive.

Keep it gentle

Vigorous massage is best avoided in all arthritic conditions.

EASING SYMPTOMS

■ Regular cups of celery seed, white willow and lignum vitae decoction in equal amounts (two teaspoons of the mix per cup) can help.

■ Alternatively, drink an infusion of stinging nettles, bogbean, meadowsweet and fennel three times a day.

■ Add chamomile or yarrow oil to infused bladderwrack oil (five drops of essential oil per teaspoon) and rub gently into affected joints.

■ Apply a poultice of chamomile flowers, hops or comfrey to painful joints.

■ Take dily supplements of devil's claw (1–2 g), evening primrose (2 g) preferably with an additional fish oil, vitamin C (1–3 g) and zinc (25 mg).

■ Apply an ice pack of frozen peas for 10 minutes each day to ease stiffness.

■ Eat a low salt diet, plenty of oily fish and minimal dairy products.

GOUT

Gout is an acutely painful diet-related condition, which is often an inherited tendency and does not always afflict the overindulgent as was once widely believed. The pain is caused by a build-up of uric acid crystals in the joints – commonly the big toe joint – associated with an inability to break down purines, a group of chemicals found in shellfish, red meats, fatty fish and offal.

celery seeds, yarrow and meadowsweet infusion

TREATMENT

■ If you suffer from gout, cut down on foods containing purines and avoid those containing large amounts of oxalic acid especially rhubarb, sorrel and spinach. Drink plenty of water and increase your intake of diuretics to flush the uric acid out of the system.

■ Make a decoction from celery seed, gravel root and black cohosh (one teaspoon of the mix per cup, three times a day) or use an infusion of meadowsweet, yarrow and celery seeds in the same way.

■ To relieve the pain of an attack, add a few drops of clove to a little warm water and use the mix to soak a compress which can then be gently applied to the affected area.

RHEUMATISM AND LUMBAGO

The muscular aches and pains labelled as "rheumatism" can have many causes. To the medical profession "rheumatic diseases" include all the various types of arthritis and gout. Lumbago is pain in the lower back, sciatica is a pain felt along the back and outer side of the thigh, leg and foot, associated with the sciatic nerve, and fibrositis is an inflammation of fibrous tissue (especially muscle sheaths) which often affects the back muscles.

TREATMENT

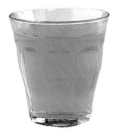

meadowsweet, yarrow and rosemary infusion

■ Use cleansing herbs to remove toxins from the system, along with anti-inflammatories and pain-killing rubs. For example, drink an infusion made from equal amounts of meadowsweet, yarrow and rosemary (one teaspoon per cup) or use celery seed and white willow as a decoction.

■ To treat rheumatism or lumbago externally add five drops of marjoram and rosemary oil to a tablespoon of almond oil, then use this to gently massage any aching areas. Infused cayenne oil can also be an effective treatment, but it can irritate sensitive skins, so use cautiously and dilute it with more almond oil if you suffer any adverse reactions.

TENNIS ELBOW AND FROZEN SHOULDER

Inflammation of the tendon at the outer edge of the elbow, usually caused by excessive exercise, is usually referred to as tennis elbow (but also as golfer's, miner's or tailor's elbow). A frozen shoulder is chronic stiffness of the shoulder joint, which usually has no obvious cause.

TREATMENT

Both tennis elbow and frozen shoulder respond to herbal anti-inflammatories applied topically. Mix 5 ml each of lavender and chamomile oil with 40 ml of infused St. John's wort, oil and store in a dark glass bottle. Use the mix to massage the elbow or shoulder frequently.

A compress soaked in dilute arnica tincture (two teaspoons to a cup of warm water) can also ease local pain.

Internally, celery seed and lignum vitae tea (see Rheumatoid arthritis, p.57) can help.

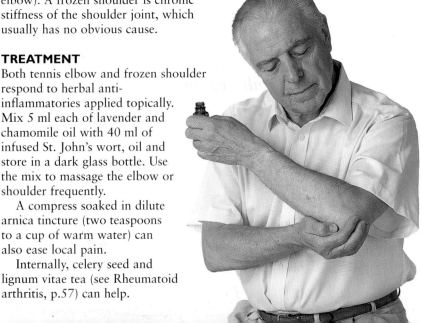

HERBS FOR THE MIND

Herbs act on many levels. They can ease physical tensions, directly affect our emotions and mental energy, and bring a spiritual dimension. In Ayurvedic tradition, many herbs are believed to improve our capacity for love and compassion, and ancient Taoists in China used certain herbs to increase their determination to lead a virtuous life.

Many European herbs also had ancient sacred connections, although these were condemned by medieval Christians: vervain, for example, was sacred to Jove and was used in Druidic rituals with spiritual aspects. Today we use the herb as a relaxing nervine (for calming the nerves), although some people still believe it has a spiritual dimension and will heal holes in the human aura.

Relaxing herb teas are ideal for everyday drinking, while Bach Flower Remedies and essential oils may be used for more direct action on our emotions.

TENSION AND STRESS

Herbal remedies have a variety of powerful effects on our mental well-being. They include sedatives to ease tensions and anxiety, remedies that act directly on the emotions, tonics and stimulants to provide additional short-term energy, and long-term energy tonics to build stamina and combat stress.

COPING WITH STRESS

Stress is an essential part of our lives and is not necessarily negative – it helps us to maintain vigour and vitality and provides a stimulus for activity and invention. When faced with a stressful situation, our bodies produce adrenaline – the "flight or fight" hormone, which prompts us to run away or strike out. Modern life does not, however, always permit us to run or fight, and we have to respond in a more socially acceptable way and suppress the adrenaline rush. This leads to a negative stress response in which the body remains over-active. When this response occurs repeatedly, it can damage our health and increase the risk of chronic illness.

SYMPTOMS
■ Palpitations (becoming aware of one's heartbeat) or possibly panic attacks.

■ Dry mouth.

■ Constant tiredness, difficulties with sleep and concentration.

■ An inability to relax.

■ Recurring headaches, muscular aches and pains, diarrhoea or stomach upsets.

■ Easy tears and a tendency to feel low – in severe cases this can lead to depressive illness.

REMEDIES
Herbs cannot solve major lifestyle problems (although they can help give us the will to make the necessary changes), but they can ease the symptoms and improve our ability to cope.

■ Siberian ginseng helps the body to cope more efficiently with stress: take up to 600 mg a day for 10–14 days before the stresses are due to peak. This can be a useful preventative before exams, a busy time at work or long-haul air travel to combat jet lag.

■ Reishi mushroom capsules can help you make necessary changes in lifestyle to combat stress – take 600 mg daily.

■ Relaxing herbs such as wood betony and chamomile can also help: use them in combination or separately in regular teas and add five drops of lavender oil to bath water as well.

lavender oil

3

PANIC ATTACKS

Characterized by increased heart rate or palpitations, breathlessness, pallor and sweating, panic attacks may be associated with specific anxieties and fears, or may happen with no apparent cause, leaving the sufferer feeling shaken and uncertain. Seek professional help for recurrent attacks. Some argue that panic attacks are linked to food intolerance and candidiasis which produces toxins that may interfere with neurotransmitters.

■ Occasional feelings of panic can be helped with drops of Dr Bach's Rescue Remedy on the tongue. Alternatively, use one drop of rose oil on a sugar lump slowly dissolved in the mouth. A drop of rose oil in a room diffuser or sniffed on a handkerchief will also help.

■ Drink a cup of wood betony and skullcap tea (one teaspoon of each per cup) and sip slowly while you concentrate on deep breathing.

ANXIETY AND TENSION

3

Herbal remedies cannot solve the problems that lead to anxiety, but they can help us to relax and improve our ability to cope with day-to-day tensions. For the profoundly anxious, however, herbal remedies should not be regarded as a substitute for professional counselling or psychotherapy.

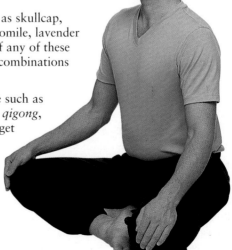

TREATMENT

■ Drink calming herbal teas such as skullcap, wood betony, lime flowers, chamomile, lavender or lemon balm. Use a teaspoon of any of these herbs per cup or try some of the combinations given on pp.108–109.

■ Learning a relaxation technique such as breath control, meditation, yoga, *qigong*, or *t'ai-chi* can help. But don't forget that is is just as important to make time to use the techniques.

■ Massage oils and Bach Flower Remedies (see p.62) can also help to ease specific problems.

BACH FLOWER REMEDIES FOR EMOTIONAL PROBLEMS

Some of the most widely available herbal remedies for the emotions are the Bach Flower Remedies, which have been used since the 1930s. In recent years, flower remedies based on American and Australian extracts have also become available. All are made up of very dilute flower extracts preserved in brandy and can be combined as necessary, then further diluted and taken in drop doses as required.

Remedy	Dr Bach's suggested use
Agrimony	Mental torture behind a "brave face"
Aspen	Vague fears of an unknown origin
Beech	Critical intolerance of others
Centaury	Weak will
Cerato	Self-doubts
Cherry Plum	Fears of mental collapse
Chestnut Bud	Refusal to learn from past mistakes
Chicory	Possessiveness and selfishness
Clematis	Inattention and dreamy escapism
Crab Apple	Feeling unclean or ashamed
Elm	Feelings of inadequacy
Gentian	Despondency and discouragement
Gorse	Hopelessness and despair
Heather	Self-centred obsession with your own troubles
Holly	Jealousy, anger or hatred of others
Honeysuckle	Homesickness and nostalgia
Hornbeam	"Monday morning feelings" and procrastination
Impatiens	Impatience
Larch	Lack of confidence
Mimulus	Fear of known things
Mustard	Deep gloom and severe depression
Oak	Struggling against adversity
Olive	Complete exhaustion
Pine	Guilt and self-blame
Red Chestnut	Excessive fear for others, especially loved ones
Rock Rose	Extreme terror
Rock Water	Overwork and refusal to relax
Scleranthus	Uncertainty and indecision
Star of Bethlehem	Shock
Sweet Chestnut	Extreme anguish; the limit of endurance
Vervain	Tension, over-enthusiasm and over-effort
Vine	Dominance and inflexibility
Walnut	Life stage transitions, as at the menopause
Water Violet	Pride and reserve
White Chestnut	Mental anguish and persistent nagging worries
Wild Oat	Uncertainty about which path to take
Wild Rose	Apathy and lack of ambition
Willow	Resentment and bitterness

3

ST. JOHN'S WORT

St. John's wort is nature's own antidepressant. Research suggests that one of the herb's active ingredients – hyperflorin – acts in much the same way as fluoxetine, a constituent of conventional pharmaceutical antidepressants.

St. John's wort is also anti-inflammatory, topically antiseptic and analgesic, and a good restorative for nervous tissues.

An infused oil (see p.34) is a useful first-aid remedy for burns, cuts and grazes, while poultices or compresses can ease neuralgia and pain following dental extractions. St. John's wort is also a traditional remedy for period pain and menopausal upsets. It contains chemicals known as hypericins which affect the immune system and have been used in AIDS therapy.

Prolonged use is said to increase the photosensitivity of the skin, although clinical evidence of this is scant.

3

DEPRESSION

Ranging from Monday morning blues to a serious clinical condition that may take years to overcome, depression should never be underestimated. Associated symptoms can include headaches, exhaustion, constipation, weight gain, menstrual irregularities, recurrent infections and lethargy. In severe cases of depression, professional help is essential.

TREATMENT

A herbal approach generally involves countering physical symptoms, such as stimulating the digestive system and strengthening the nervous system. A general anti-depressive tea could include equal amounts of damiana, lemon balm and St. John's wort (two teaspoons of the mix per cup, three or four times daily). Add skullcap if relaxation is a problem and wood betony if tension headaches are involved.

■ Many foods and culinary herbs are also anti-depressive – eat plenty of oats in porridge and use basil in cooking to help lift the spirits.

■ Take ginseng or St. John's wort tablets or capsules.

■ Bach Flower Remedies, such as gentian, gorse or mustard, may also be helpful.

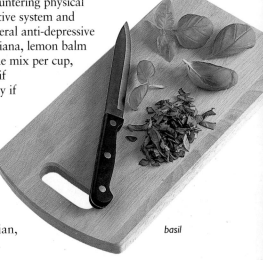

basil

EASING EXHAUSTION

Exhaustion has become one of the characteristic ills of our age: it is one of the most common reasons for seeking medical treatment while a general lack of energy can interfere with enjoyment and performance. Long hours spent working and commuting are partly to blame, as are growing pollution levels and chemical additives in our food, adding to the hidden stresses on our body systems.

TIREDNESS AND FATIGUE

It is normal to feel tired after exertion. Tiredness becomes a problem only when you start feeling exhausted after normal activities, find it difficult to concentrate, have difficulties in getting out of bed in the morning, or lack energy and the motivation to get tasks finished.

STIMULANTS

There are plenty of herbal stimulants to choose from. Coffee, tea, cola drinks and chocolate are rich in caffeine, theobromine and related alkaloids and can act as a short-term restorative. However, longer-term tonics (see pp.104–5) which help to strengthen our inner energy levels and build up our reserves are far better. Rosemary and damiana have a tonic and restorative action: make a tea containing equal amounts (one teaspoon per cup) and drink as required. The Indian herb gotu kola is equally beneficial and could be added to the mix. Rosemary, sandalwood or thyme oil added to bath water (five drops) are also stimulating.

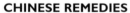

gotu kola

CHINESE REMEDIES

Chinese herbs can also be helpful. As a general energy tonic, ginseng is best taken in periods of up to four weeks, preferably as autumn gives way to winter. In China it is considered to be particularly suitable for older people and for men rather than women. However, in younger men it can give a disproportionate boost to *yang* energy levels, leading to aggression and irritation.

Rather gentler are American ginseng and codonopsis root (*dang shen*), while *dang gui* (Chinese angelica root) has long been a favourite energy tonic with Chinese women.

All of these herbs are becoming more readily available in over-the-counter preparations in the West. Take a daily dose of up to 600 mg of any of them.

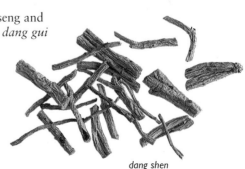

dang shen

CHRONIC FATIGUE SYNDROME

This prolonged and clinical exhaustion has been variously called neurasthenia, sick building syndrome, post-viral fatigue and myalgic encephalomyelitis (ME). Symptoms can include muscle fatigue and weakness after even minor exertion, as well as headaches, dizziness, chest pains, sleep disturbances, sore throats, breathing problems, swollen glands, recurrent infections and digestive disturbances. The problem can continue for months, or even years, and then vanish as mysteriously as it appeared.

TREATMENT

■ Strengthen the immune system with echinacea, garlic, reishi or astragalus supplements, taking two 200 mg capsules up to four times a day.

■ Use cleansing herbs to clear toxins from the tissues: process a large bowl of fresh cleavers in a food blender and take 10 ml of the juice three times daily.

■ Make an infusion containing equal amounts of gotu kola, St. John's wort and fenugreek seeds and drink a cup three times daily.

■ Daily dietary supplements should include evening primrose oil (500 mg), vitamin C (500 mg), vitamin E (400 i.u.), zinc and magnesium.

3

DEBILITY AND CONVALESCENCE

A lack of vitality and general weakness following illness is not uncommon although causes such as under-nourishment, low blood pressure or anaemia can lead to general debility at other times. Seek professional help if there seems to be no obvious reason for the problem.

TREATMENT

Eat a healthy diet with a good mineral and vitamin content – boost it with a multi-vitamin or general purpose mineral supplement if necessary. Eat plenty of alfalfa to increase vitamin and mineral intake – add the sprouted seeds to salads and sandwiches or make an infusion of the seeds (one teaspoon per cup) and drink regularly.

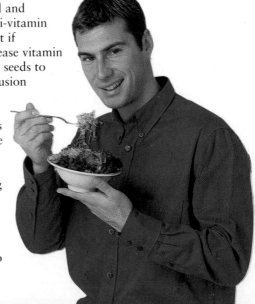

An infusion made of equal amounts of agrimony, oat straw and chamomile flowers (two teaspoons per cup, three times a day) will help; or try a decoction of equal amounts of ginseng root, liquorice root and ginger with half as much gentian root (one teaspoon of the mix per cup, three times a day). These herbs can also be taken in capsules or tablet form (up to 600 mg daily).

USING ESSENTIAL OILS AND MASSAGE

Essential oils can have a direct effect on the emotions and mental energy; combined with massage, they can help combat a range of conditions including fatigue and stress.

Although it is easy to massage your own temples and neck to combat headaches, or abdomen for period pain or digestive upsets, it is usually better to ask someone else to do it. Use oil when massaging the skin to avoid soreness from friction.

Dilute essential oils as they can irritate the skin. In most cases use five drops of oil in a teaspoon of a carrier oil such as almond or wheatgerm oil. You can mix larger amounts, using 5 ml of essential oil with 20 ml of carrier oil. Store in a clean dark glass bottle for up to three months.

Pour a little oil onto your hand and then massage this into the shoulders or back with a gentle circular motion before applying more pressure.

Among the oils most suitable for stress and fatigue problems are:

■ Basil, bergamot, chamomile, camphor, jasmine, lavender, melissa, neroli, patchouli, rose and sandalwood to help combat melancholy.

■ Basil, peppermint and rosemary to help combat fatigue.

■ Benzoin, chamomile, jasmine, lavender, marjoram, melissa, neroli, rose and sandalwood to help ease anxiety.

3

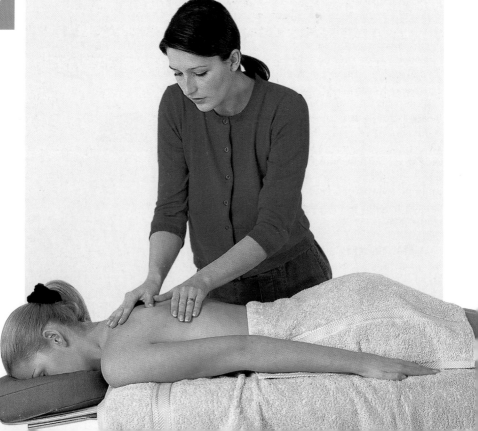

SLEEPING SOUNDLY

Whether it is a failure to get off to sleep in the first place as thoughts continue to race through the wakeful mind, or that sort of very light, easily disturbed sleep which brings restlessness in the early hours, sleeplessness is a frustrating and sometimes deeply disturbing problem which most people experience at some time or other. Fortunately, herbal remedies can very often help.

INSOMNIA

Waking restlessly in the night may be due to a failure to relax – an inability to "switch off" or a nagging preoccupation with day-to-day troubles – although it can be symptomatic of other health problems.

The Chinese consider that the body's essential energy, or *qi*, travels through all the organs at night in a regular pattern. Always waking at a particular time might suggest an imbalance in a particular system or organ. Noting the waking time is a good idea in order to see if a pattern emerges and track down the source of the problem.

Waking up in order to urinate is another common problem – try limiting your fluid intake in the evening, or seek professional help if a urinary or kidney problem may be to blame.

Relaxing before bedtime can help with sleeplessness – try a hot bath with a few drops of lavender, chamomile or basil oil added, or spend a few minutes sitting calmly and concentrating on your breathing.

The herbs discussed below can be helpful taken regularly in night-time teas (see also Chamomile, p.109; Lemon Balm, p.96), used singly or mixed with wood betony, St. John's wort or lavender. Use one or two teaspoons of the herb or herb combination per cup. It is best to vary your remedy frequently because constant use can reduce efficacy.

CALIFORNIAN POPPY
Although it is a member of the poppy family, this American plant – which is known locally as nightcap – contains none of the potent alkaloids normally associated with the family, so is quite safe and non-addictive.

Californian poppies are annual and easy to grow in Europe. To use them in herbal remedies, collect the entire plant towards the end of the flowering period. Dry the poppies in small bunches (5–6 stems), then crumble the leaves, flowers and stems and store in airtight jars ready for use in home-made remedies.

lavender

HOPS

Although we tend to associate hops mainly with beer, to which they give the characteristic bitter flavour, it wasn't until the 17th century that they were used in brewing. Hops also help to stimulate the digestion.

The volatile oils in hops are sedative and soporific – hence their popular use in herbal sleep pillows. Hop oils evaporate over time, so the hops should be replaced in the pillow every few months to maintain its efficacy.

The herb can also be taken as an infusion to aid sleep – add some honey to make it more palatable.

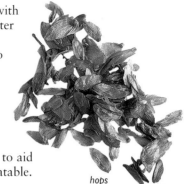
hops

PASSIONFLOWER

A symbolic association with Christianity, rather than any likely effect on our emotions, gives these flowers their name. Far from provoking excitement, this herb is actually a potent sedative which relaxes the nerves and relieves stress, making it likely to ensure a good night's sleep. Use it in an infusion or take 20 drops of the tincture at night. Passionflower is best taken for no more than 10–14 days at a time with breaks of three or four days in between. It should not be taken during pregnancy because it may act as a uterine stimulant.

3

LIME FLOWERS

Linden or lime flowers have been a traditional European remedy for over-excitement and nervous upsets for centuries. They are very soothing and can be used for easing stress as well as in an evening drink.

Linden is also used to help with high blood pressure problems and can reduce the damage associated with atherosclerosis (see p.47). The taste can be a little bland – add a pinch of peppermint to the infusion to improve it.

WILD LETTUCE

Until the 1930s, the thick latex-like sap of this soporific plant was collected, dried and sold by chemists as "lettuce opium" – a potent but non-addictive sedative.

The dried herb can be made into an infusion to be drunk at bedtime. Alternatively, take 10–20 drops of wild lettuce tincture in half a glass or less of water before going to bed.

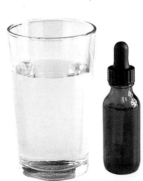
wild lettuce tincture

NERVE AND TENSION PAIN

Among the most common results of stress and nervous upsets are tension headaches and migraine attacks. Although many people suffer when they are obviously under pressure, whether at home or at work, others find that their symptoms worsen when they start to relax – Saturday morning migraines are common among those who work hard all week and start to unwind on Friday night.

TENSION HEADACHES

If a headache starts with a tightening of the muscles at the back of the neck followed by muscle spasm spreading forward across the scalp, it is probably due to stress or nervous tension. However, this type of headache can also be caused by sitting or working awkwardly for long periods. Days spent hunched at a desk or over a computer keyboard can be a source of tension headache.

REMEDIES
■ Massage the nape of the neck and temples with two or three drops each of lavender, juniper and thyme oils in two teaspoons of almond oil in order to relieve muscle spasms and prevent the headache developing.

3

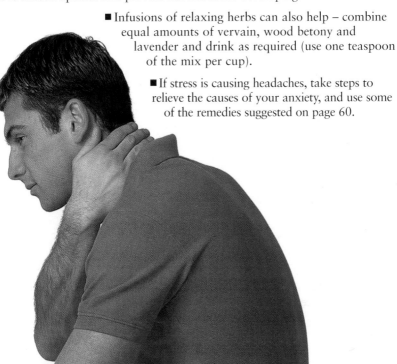

■ Infusions of relaxing herbs can also help – combine equal amounts of vervain, wood betony and lavender and drink as required (use one teaspoon of the mix per cup).

■ If stress is causing headaches, take steps to relieve the causes of your anxiety, and use some of the remedies suggested on page 60.

NEURALGIA

Sharp, shooting pains travelling along the route of a nerve are usually described as neuralgia. The problem usually involves inflammation of the nerve fibres and can occur anywhere, although it is most common along the trigeminal nerve, which runs along the side of the face and scalp. The pain is often exacerbated by cold and draughts – common triggers include going out on windy days with damp hair, and exercising out of doors in cold weather.

REMEDIES

Herbalists treat this condition with a combination of nerve tonics such as vervain, skullcap or St. John's wort; painkillers; circulatory stimulants such as ginger and cayenne; and sedatives.

■ Make an infusion containing equal amounts of vervain or skullcap and St. John's wort (one or two teaspoons per cup) and add a pinch of powdered ginger or cayenne or a clove before drinking.

■ Application of lemon oil, lavender oil or infused St. John's wort oil to the affected area may also help to relieve the symptoms – add five drops of lemon oil to a teaspoon of warm water, or use the lavender and St. John's wort combination suggested for burns (see p.33). (Warmed slices of fresh lemon or lemon juice mixed with warm water make a good substitute for lemon oil.)

■ Alternatively, apply a warm compress that has been soaked in St. John's wort, lavender or vervain infusion to the affected area.

3

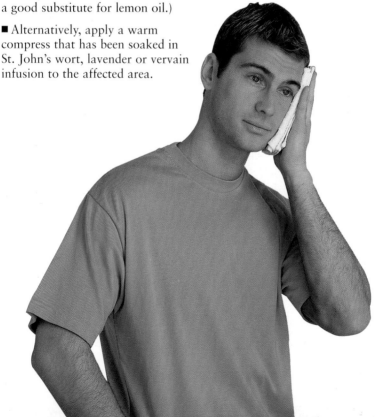

MIGRAINE

There are two categories of migraine – classical and common. Both types start with visual disturbances, typically jagged lights at the edge of the visual field. Sufferers may also experience pins-and-needles in the hands and a characteristic metallic taste in the mouth.

In classic migraine the symptoms usually subside within a few minutes but in common migraine they are inevitably followed by a severe headache and increased sensitivity to light. There may also be nausea and vomiting. Sufferers usually need to lie down in a darkened room until the attack eases – this may take a few hours but in severe cases it can run into days.

Frequent bilious attacks in a child can often be a precursor of migraine in later life. Recent research has suggested that migraine sufferers under 45 have an increased risk of stroke.

Persistent or sudden unusually severe headaches lasting for three days or more should be referred to a medical practitioner.

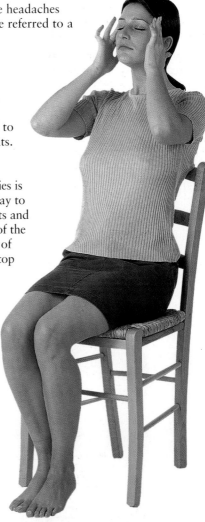

CAUSES
Migraine is often associated with food intolerance, usually involving red wine, chocolate, pork, citrus fruits, coffee or cheese. The problem can also be linked to stress or the strobic effect of bright lights.

REMEDIES
■ One of the most popular herbal remedies is feverfew. Try chewing a fresh leaf each day to prevent attacks, or use ready-made tablets and capsules. Feverfew can cause ulceration of the mucous membranes (usually in the form of mouth ulcers) in sensitive individuals – stop taking it immediately if this happens.

■ Massaging dilute lavender oil (20 drops in one teaspoon of almond oil) into the temples can sometimes help prevent an attack developing.

■ During an attack, sip an infusion containing equal amounts of lavender, wood betony and St. John's wort (two teaspoons of the mix per cup).

■ Valerian tablets may also help.

■ Yellow jasmine and Jamaican dogwood are potent remedies, but sale of these is restricted and they need to be prescribed by a herbalist.

OLD AGE

The "third age" brings its own health problems. The body shows signs of wear and tear, and often short-term memory starts to fade – while recall of childhood events may be impressive, many old people find it difficult to remember what they did a few hours before.

CONFUSION

Confusion in the elderly may be associated with senile dementia, but it can also be linked to a hardening of the cerebral arteries and a reduced blood supply to the brain.

ginkgo

Impressive results have been claimed for ginkgo, which improves cerebral circulation. It is available as liquid extracts and tablets. Simply use two or three fresh leaves per cup in an infusion. Wood betony has a similar action on the brain's blood supply. Use it in infusions (one teaspoon per cup) or tinctures (5 ml or one teaspoon three times a day), or combine with half as much European periwinkle (not the Madagascan variety, which is toxic), which also helps to combat hardening of the cerebral arteries.

FAILING MEMORY

Herbs are not a panacea for memory loss, but they can help older people to remain alert and active and provide a gentle boost to concentration and memory.

Sage and rosemary, two of the many herbs traditionally believed to improve the memory, are now known to be powerful antioxidants which can combat cell decay and destroy free radicals – groups of atoms from our food which scavenge among our cells for oxygen.

Drink cups of sage or rosemary infusion (one teaspoon per cup) instead of tea or coffee or use *gotu kola*, which is equally rejuvenating. Use rosemary oil as a massage or add a couple of drops to a room diffuser to scent the house.

GINKGO

The ginkgo tree is a rare fossil survivor – a deciduous conifer which has been unchanged since before the evolution of mammals. The seeds have been used for centuries in traditional Chinese medicine to treat asthma and urinary problems, but in the past few years Western researchers have also found that the plant significantly improves the circulation. In Germany, ginkgo has been successfully used to speed the recovery of patients after brain surgery. Its strong effect on the cerebral circulation has led many to regard it as an anti-ageing remedy, since hardening of the cerebral arteries is a common cause of apparent confusion in the elderly.

HERBS FOR MEN AND WOMEN

Herbs have been used for centuries to cope with a wide range of human reproductive disorders: simple analgesics to soothe period pains, uterine stimulants in childbirth or aphrodisiacs to help with sexual dysfunction.

Clinical trials have demonstrated that many of these remedies do affect hormonal function. Chaste-tree, for example, stimulates female hormone production so was used by medieval monks as an anaphrodisiac. Sage bolsters oestrogen levels, explaining its traditional role as an energy tonic for older women.

Other cultures put less emphasis on hormones than on inherent energy levels: traditional Chinese theory maintains that our reproductive energies gradually run down during our lives and explains many symptoms of ageing – from hearing loss to the menopause – in terms of this declining energy.

MENSTRUAL PROBLEMS

The monthly menstrual cycle starts with menstruation, when the lining of the uterus is shed. This is followed by the release of a new egg from the ovaries about two weeks later. The uterus lining thickens again until around day 26 when the unfertilized egg is shed, followed by the uterus lining, beginning menstruation once more. Throughout the cycle, the female sex hormones, oestrogen and progesterone, follow a pattern of increasing and decreasing levels. For most women this cycle proceeds with little change – pregnancies excepted – for 30 to 40 years. Herbal remedies can help with common problems, such as period pain, and can support professional treatment in more serious conditions too.

PREMENSTRUAL SYNDROME (PMS)

PMS is a term for a range of cyclical irregularities that can include abdominal bloating, emotional disturbances, food cravings, palpitations, fluid retention, headaches, vaginal discharge and breast tenderness.

REMEDIES

■ Among the most popular herbal remedies are chaste-tree, often sold as agnus-castus (See p.83), and evening primrose oil, which contains an essential fatty acid (*gamma*-linolenic acid). Borage and blackcurrant seed oils, also available commercially, contain the same fatty acid. Take 500 mg daily of any of these oils in capsules; increase to 1 g daily in the ten days before a period is due.

■ Traditional Chinese medicine links menstruation with liver function and focuses on toning this organ using herbs such as *dang gui*.

4

■ Suitable herbal teas may also help. Try a decoction of equal amounts of chaste-tree berries, false unicorn root and black cohosh (one teaspoon of the mix per cup). An alternative is an infusion of equal amounts of vervain, yarrow and sage (one teaspoon of the mix per cup). Drink up to four cups a day in the ten days before the period starts (or from 19 days after a period if that is easier to count).

■ Drops of chaste-tree tincture taken in water each morning can also help – use ten drops increasing to 20 drops in the ten days before the period is due.

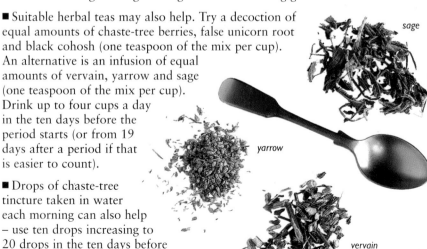

sage

yarrow

vervain

BREAST DISCOMFORT AND BENIGN LUMPS

Painful and swollen breasts are a common symptom of PMS – some women even find they have to wear a larger size of bra just before a period.

Lumpiness in the breasts may also become pronounced in the days before a period. Breast lumps are often associated with fibrocystic breast disease (FBD), in which numerous small hard, benign cysts form. While there are often no other symptoms, the condition can be associated with sluggish liver function and poor circulation – there may be a tendency for varicose veins, piles or chilblains as well. Symptoms usually get worse in the few days before a period. FBD sufferers should carry out regular breast self-examination and be alert for any change in the lumps.

REMEDIES

■ If premenstrual breast pain is a regular problem, add a few pieces of bitter orange or tangerine peel to one of the PMS teas suggested opposite.

■ Apply a compress soaked in horsetail and cleavers infusion to help relieve severe discomfort.

■ Liver-stimulating herbs can help – make a decoction of burdock and dandelion roots with an equal amount of hawthorn berries. Use one to two teaspoons in all per cup and add a pinch of powdered ginger.

■ Alternatively, try an infusion containing equal amounts of vervain, cleavers and lady's mantle (two teaspoons per cup, three times daily).

■ Take 1 g of evening primrose oil in capsules daily.

4

PERIOD PAIN

Painful periods are accepted by many women as quite normal – though they need not be. Herbalists tend to divide period pain into two types:

■ Congestive pain, which builds up shortly before the period starts and is associated with blood stagnation; it may also involve abdominal bloating and fluid retention and generally eases once bleeding starts.

■ Spasmodic pain, caused by muscle cramps in the uterus as it sheds its lining; this usually starts with bleeding and may last for one or two days.

REMEDIES

■ As a general-purpose remedy, mix equal amounts of St. John's wort, raspberry leaf and yarrow (one teaspoon per cup of infusion) and drink as required while symptoms last. For congestive pain, add a teaspoon of vervain and motherwort; for spasmodic pain, add chamomile and pasque flower.

■ All types of period pain will respond to massage – mix five drops each of rosemary and basil oils in a teaspoon of almond oil and massage the area between the navel and pubic bone

■ For spasmodic pain, a simple remedy is to take 20–25 ml of black haw tincture in half a glass of warm water when the pain starts. One dose is often quite enough to solve the problem.

■ Between periods, drink raspberry leaf and yarrow tea as a tonic for the uterus and reproductive system (do not take these herbs if you are trying to conceive). Chaste-tree tincture used as for PMS (see p.74) will help to normalize hormonal function.

HEAVY PERIODS

While fibroids (see below) are a common cause of excessive menstrual bleeding, very often there is no pathological explanation. Some women always have heavy periods and many just accept the resulting risk of anaemia and exhaustion as quite normal. Herbs can often help, although it is important to seek medical advice if the pattern of monthly flow changes significantly.

TREATMENT

Shepherd's purse (also known as mother's hearts), American cranesbill, periwinkle, white deadnettle, raspberry leaf, marigold and lady's mantle may all be used in decoctions or infusions – combine equal amounts of shepherd's purse, lady's mantle and raspberry leaf, for example, and take two cups daily; increase to four cups during menstruation. You can also use any of these herbs as alternatives to tea and coffee drinks throughout the day.

To avoid anaemia, eat plenty of iron-rich foods (such as red meat, watercress, apricots and blackcurrants) and herbs (such as nettles and parsley) and take two 200 mg capsules of *dang gui* daily.

4

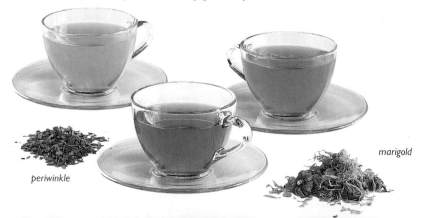

marigold

periwinkle

FIBROIDS

Heavy menstrual bleeding is often the only sign of fibroids, which are benign growths in the uterus. Usually there is no pain, although large fibroids may cause painful intercourse. The presence of fibroids may affect fertility. As oestrogen levels fall after the menopause, most fibroids will shrink naturally.

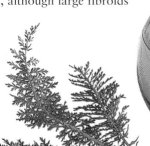

TREATMENT

The usual orthodox solution is surgery. Herbal treatment can be successful but may work slowly, so give it time to show results and don't be rushed into the surgical option.

Professional herbal treatment is advisable but simple home remedies include regular infusions using equal amounts of periwinkle, marigold, lady's mantle and cleavers (two teaspoons per cup, three times daily). Take ten drops of chaste-tree tincture in water each morning as well. If heavy menstrual bleeding is a problem, drink yarrow and shepherd's purse tea as well.

Maintain as healthy a diet as possible, stop taking oral contraceptives and avoid foods rich in organic sterols (hormone-like substances) – these include many members of the bean family.

RASPBERRY LEAF

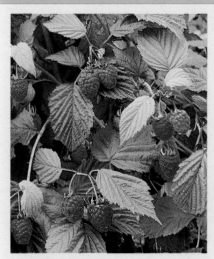

Raspberry leaf, well known as a *partus praeparator* (preparation for childbirth) is used in the weeks before birth to help prepare the uterus for labour. It is also a uterine relaxant, astringent and tonic so is helpful for period pain and heavy bleeding.

Its astringent action also makes raspberry leaf ideal for inflamed mucous membranes – such as a gargle for sore throats and in infusions to ease the discomfort of diarrhoea.

To use as a preparation for labour, start taking raspberry leaf tea once or twice a day no sooner than eight weeks before the estimated due date and continue sipping cups of it during labour.

4

PREGNANCY AND BIRTH

For generations women depended solely on herbs to ease the ills of pregnancy and the trauma of childbirth. Today modern medicine has made this once high-risk stage in a woman's life much safer, but traditional remedies can still have a part to play. As with other forms of medication, take no more than is necessary and limit treatment to as short a time as possible. Avoid taking any unnecessary medication during the first three months of pregnancy and consult the list of herbs to avoid on page 81 before taking any over-the-counter products.

MINOR ILLS OF PREGNANCY

As well as the ailments covered here, see Iron-deficient anaemia, p.46; Cystitis, p.88; Cramp, p.30; Coping with stress, p.60; Fainting, p.30; Insomnia, p.67; Piles, p.49; Thrush, p.83; Varicose veins, p.49.

BACKACHE
Add five drops of lavender oil or a cup of strained chamomile infusion to a bath for pain relief, or use the same oils for massage (two or three drops of either in a teaspoon of almond oil or infused St. John's wort): add one drop of ginger or black pepper oil to the mix if the pain is particularly acute. Drink an infusion containing St. John's wort and chamomile (one teaspoon of each per cup) three times daily.

chamomile

St. John's wort

FATIGUE
Tiredness may indicate iron-deficient anaemia – routine antenatal blood tests should pick this up. For general use take Siberian ginseng (up to 600 mg daily) for up to a month to provide an energy boost. Extended use of Korean ginseng is best avoided.

CONSTIPATION
Ensure that there is enough fibre in the diet by eating plenty of fresh apples and lightly cooked vegetables. Ispaghula husks or seeds (see p.53) are ideal; avoid strong purgatives like senna, alder buckthorn (also known as frangula bark) and cascara sagrada, as the excessive gut spasm they cause may irritate the uterus. Instead, opt for milder remedies such as dandelion root, butternut or liquorice (one teaspoon of the mixture per cup of decoction each morning); add a pinch of powdered ginger or crushed fennel seeds to ease any discomfort from griping pains.

HEARTBURN AND INDIGESTION

Eat slowly, taking frequent small meals rather than two or three large ones a day, and avoid coffee and fatty or spicy foods. Gentle indigestion remedies are ideal – try a cup of catmint, lemon balm or chamomile infusion after meals. Fennel and spearmint can be used occasionally in the same way but large doses should be avoided in pregnancy. Chew slippery elm tablets or take a gruel before meals (see p.27).

MORNING SICKNESS

Ginger is one of the best herbs to use and doses of up to 1 g can be quite safe. Also recommended are bitter orange, black horehound, fennel, lemon balm, chamomile and peppermint. Vary the remedy for best results. Dilute tinctures of each herb with an equal amount of water and store in separate dropper bottles; then take four or five drops of one of the remedies on the tongue before rising or at the first sign of nausea. Change your preferred herb every few days. Alternatively, use infusions or decoctions of any of these herbs (half a cup at a time).

CHILDBIRTH

While herbs once played a key role in childbirth, stimulating contractions, easing labour and helping to expel the placenta, modern medicine has largely superseded these traditional remedies. Nevertheless, herbs can still be of use.

4

PREPARING FOR LABOUR

Many women take raspberry leaf tea (see p.77) to help strengthen the uterus. A daily cup of motherwort tea in the final weeks will help to calm the nerves.

DURING LABOUR

During the first stage of labour, sip a cup of infusion made from equal amounts of rose petals, wood betony and raspberry leaves (two teaspoons of the mixture per cup). Massage the lower back, abdomen and inner thighs with a mix of ten drops each of lavender and jasmine in two tablespoons almond or olive oil. A hot compress soaked in marigold, mugwort or wood betony infusion applied to the lower abdomen above the pubic area will also help.

AFTER THE BIRTH

Immediately after the birth, start to take homoeopathic Arnica 6X tablets (one every 15–30 minutes for several hours) to repair bruised and torn tissues and speed recovery from the shock of the birth.

BREAST-FEEDING

Many herbs will stimulate milk flow – drink regular cups of fennel, dill, caraway or anise to boost milk production and deliver a suitable carminative to combat colic in the baby at the same time. Other suitable milk stimulants include vervain, nettles, basil, raspberry leaf, fenugreek, milk thistle, borage and goat's rue. The specific breast-feeding problems listed below respond to herbal remedies.

ENGORGEMENT
When the breasts are over-full with milk and so become swollen and tender, they are said to be engorged. Commonest in the first five days after the birth, engorgement is simply eased by expressing some of the surplus milk by hand. A warm compress soaked in lavender or chamomile infusion applied to the breast will encourage milk flow during the process. At weaning, any excess milk production can be eased by drinking two to three cups of sage infusion each day.

MASTITIS
This inflammation of the breast tissue can be very painful, with the risk of feverish symptoms which may need antibiotic treatment. The traditional solution is to insert a crushed cabbage leaf between bra and breast; replace the leaf every four hours. A poultice of common plantain leaves makes a good alternative.

4

SORE NIPPLES
This is the commonest reason for giving up breast-feeding. It is often due to poor positioning of the baby, who needs to suck over the entire areola not just the nipple. Treat by applying marigold or chamomile cream to the areola after each feed.

Cracked nipples can be a sign of yeast infection and are common if the baby is suffering from oral thrush. Marigold or tea tree can give temporary relief, although it is more important to clear the baby's infection.

Warning

Some herbs can stimulate the uterus, causing premature contractions and increasing the risk of miscarriage, while others contain toxic chemicals which may cross the placenta and enter the foetus' blood supply, leading to damage. Check with a professional herbalist if you are in doubt. (Botanical names are given for those plants not mentioned elsewhere or listed on pp.6–8.)

Avoid entirely

Alder buckthorn
Aloe
Autumn crocus (Colichicum autumnale)
Barberry
Basil oil
Beth root (Trillium erectum)
Black cohosh
Blue cohosh (Caulophyllum thalictroides)
Cascara sagrada
Comfrey
Clove oil
Cowslip
Dang gui
Devil's claw
False unicorn root (Chamaelirium luteum)
Feverfew
Golden seal (Hydrastis canadensis)
Greater celandine
Juniper
Lady's mantle
Liferoot (Senecio aureus)
Mistletoe (Viscum album)
Mugwort
Pennyroyal (Mentha pulegium)
Pokeroot (Phytolacca decandra)
Pasque flower
Rhubarb root
Rue (Ruta graveolens)
Sassafras (Sassafras albidum)
Senna
Shepherd's purse
Southernwood (Artemisia abrotanum)
Squill (Urginea maritima)
Tansy (Tanacetum vulgare)
Thuja
Wild yam
Wormwood

Use in moderation

These herbs are safe in culinary quantities or in drop doses of tincture, in the final weeks of pregnancy or during labour. The list also includes some essential oils to avoid though the herbs they are derived from are safe:

Angelica
Anise and aniseed oil
Bitter orange
Caraway
Cayenne
Chamomile oil
Celery seed (Apium graveolens)
Cinnamon (Cinnamomum zeylanicum)
Fennel
Fenugreek
Garlic
Gotu kola
Jasmine oil
Korean ginseng
Lavender
Liquorice
Lovage (Levisticum officinale)
Marjoram
Motherwort
Myrrh
Nutmeg (Myristica fragrans)
Oregano (Origanum X marjoricum; O. onites)
Parsley
Passionflower
Peppermint oil
Raspberry leaf
Rosemary and rosemary oil
Saffron (Crocus sativa)
Sage and sage oil
Thyme oil
Vervain
White horehound (Marrubium vulgare)
Wood betony
Yarrow (Achillea millefolium)

4

MENOPAUSAL PROBLEMS

While in the West we regard the menopause as related purely to changing hormonal levels at the end of a woman's reproductive life, the Chinese see it in terms of a decrease in the essential "reproductive energy" which is stored in the kidneys, and treat menopausal problems with plenty of warming kidney tonics.

HOT FLUSHES AND NIGHT SWEATS

These typical symptoms involve a sudden hot feeling across the face or body – despite the names, there is rarely any obvious redness or excess sweating.

REMEDIES
Try infusions containing an equal amount of sage, mugwort and vervain (one to two teaspoons per cup, three or four times daily), or take a high dose of evening primrose or borage oil (up to 3 g a day). Chaste-tree can also help – take 20 drops of tincture in water morning and evening. If hot flushes are accompanied by palpitations, add an equal amount of motherwort to the infusion.

EMOTIONAL UPSETS

Mood swings, depression, insomnia and anxiety can accompany the menopause and are generally attributed to hormonal changes.

REMEDIES
■ Drink suitable herbal teas, especially vervain, wood betony, lemon balm and skullcap – make an infusion containing equal amounts of wood betony and lemon balm, for example. Use up to two teaspoons of mixed herbs per cup and drink up to four cups daily.

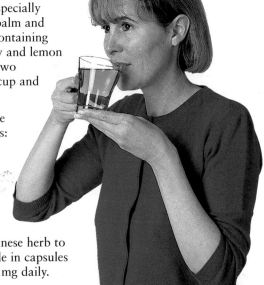

■ To the above mixture, add the following for specific symptoms: St. John's wort for depression; lime flowers for anxiety and tension; motherwort for palpitations; rose petals for panic attacks; or rosemary for poor memory.

■ *He shou wu* is a popular Chinese herb to boost kidney energies. Available in capsules and tinctures – take up to 600 mg daily.

CHASTE-TREE

Chaste-tree berries – often sold as agnus-castus – act on the pituitary gland to increase the production of the female hormones involved in ovulation. This makes the herb extremely useful for menstrual irregularities and menopausal problems. The plant reputedly takes its name from its action as a male anaphrodisiac, it was used by medieval monks to reduce libido, although some maintain that the white flowers were a symbol of female virginity. The tree grows naturally in Mediterranean regions and in Greece the berries are used as a female aphrodisiac.

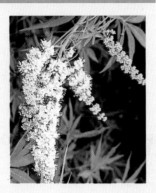

FLUID RETENTION

Commonly associated with hormonal change during menstruation, pregnancy or the menopause, fluid retention can cause symptoms ranging from abdominal bloating to severe swelling in ankles and legs with palpitations and headaches. Fluid retention can indicate diabetes or heart disorders, so seek professional help for sudden onset or a changed pattern of symptoms.

REMEDIES
■ Make an infusion of equal amounts of parsley, dandelion leaf and yarrow (two teaspoons per cup) and drink up to three cups a day. Add half as much motherwort to the mix if palpitations are also a problem.

■ For fluid retention in pregnancy avoid parsley and yarrow – instead purée a handful of fresh cleavers. Take 1 tablespoon in water, up to three times a day.

4

VAGINAL ITCHING, DRYNESS AND THRUSH

As the tissues of the vagina age and lose their elasticity (atrophic vaginitis) dryness and itching can be a problem. Changes in the natural bacterial population can also lead to an increased risk of thrush. Itching can be a symptom of both thrush and atrophic vaginitis.

■ Regular sexual intercourse will keep the vaginal walls supple and healthy and maintain their natural lubricating secretions.

■ If dryness is a problem, use a little marigold cream or a proprietary lubricant (such as K-Y Jelly).

■ Treat thrush with tea tree pessaries or put a few drops of tea tree oil on a tampon and insert into the vagina. Leave for three to four hours and repeat the process three or four times daily. Calendula and tea tree creams can be used instead, or try lady's mantle cream with a few drops of rose oil.

INFERTILITY

Infertility and lack of libido can be a problem for both men and women, putting significant strain on a relationship and leading in some cases to emotional problems. A healthy diet, relaxed approach to life and minimal contact with pollutants are essential. Studies have shown that male infertility is commonly associated with oestrogen-like pollutants in drinking water, while women trying to combine a full-time career with motherhood often find it very difficult to conceive.

MALE INFERTILITY

As well as pollutants and pesticides, low sperm count can be associated with junk food and oestrogen-mimicking chemicals in household detergents. Sperm need to be kept cool to stay fully active, so tight, hot underwear and trousers can easily contribute to infertility problems.

REMEDIES

Herbs to help improve male fertility include Korean ginseng, gotu kola, damiana and saw palmetto. Make an infusion containing equal amounts of gotu kola and damiana (two teaspoons per cup) and drink three times daily, or use saw palmetto or ginseng in capsules (up to 600 mg daily). If stress is a contributing factor, drink one or two cups of skullcap, vervain or chamomile infusion daily.

FEMALE INFERTILITY

Modern fertilization techniques can be very successful, but they are often invasive, require dedication by both partners and do not guarantee success.

CAUSES AND TREATMENT

■ Stress can be a significant factor, so use relaxing herbal teas (such as chamomile, lemon balm, wood betony, skullcap or vervain) and cut out alcohol, which can also interfere with conception.

■ Many women find it difficult to conceive after taking the oral contraceptive pill so be prepared to wait for a year or two after stopping. Chaste-tree berries will help to stimulate female hormone production and normalize ovulation (take 20 drops of tincture each morning). In addition, make an infusion containing equal amounts of red clover flowers, stinging nettles, peppermint, motherwort and marigold petals and drink a cup (two teaspoons per cup) three times daily.

■ The Chinese herb *dang gui* is also an effective tonic for the female reproductive organs. Take up to 600 mg in capsules each day on the ten days following each period, but only if there is no chance that you may be pregnant.

skullcap tea

LOSS OF LIBIDO

Stress, overwork, alcohol and excess caffeine can all contribute to problems with libido – exhaustion in particular is an effective barrier to normal sexual relations. The rhythm of the menstrual cycle also plays its part – women often feel more enthusiastic mid-cycle, just prior to ovulation, and again before menstruation when pressure from the thick endometrium stimulates sexual activity.

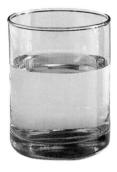 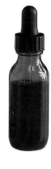

REMEDIES FOR WOMEN

For women, 20 drops of chaste-tree tincture in a little water each morning will not only stimulate the reproductive system but will also have an aphrodisiac effect. If exhaustion and overwork are a problem, drinking an infusion containing equal amounts of raspberry leaf, rosemary, motherwort and gotu kola up to three times a day will provide a stimulating tonic for the entire system.

REMEDIES FOR MEN

For many men, doubts about their performance are enough to prevent satisfactory erection and orgasm, or the problem may be more mundane – painful piles are a common cause of impotence.

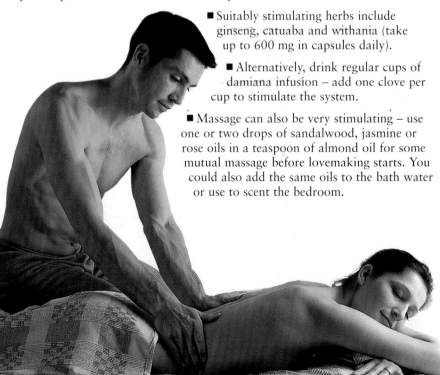

- Suitably stimulating herbs include ginseng, catuaba and withania (take up to 600 mg in capsules daily).

- Alternatively, drink regular cups of damiana infusion – add one clove per cup to stimulate the system.

- Massage can also be very stimulating – use one or two drops of sandalwood, jasmine or rose oils in a teaspoon of almond oil for some mutual massage before lovemaking starts. You could also add the same oils to the bath water or use to scent the bedroom.

4

PROSTATE PROBLEMS

The prostate gland is one of the male sex organs, found just below the bladder with an opening into the urethra. It produces an alkaline fluid which is contained in semen and is a common source of health problems, especially in older men. The situation is often made worse because men tend to be reluctant to seek help for health problems. As a result, prostate cancer often goes undiagnosed with fatal consequences.

PROSTATE ENLARGEMENT

The prostate gland often enlarges in older men, causing bladder problems; usual symptoms are a reduced urine flow with a tendency for dribbling and a need to empty the bladder at night. Residual urine often remains in the bladder where it can cause infection, or may travel back from the bladder to the kidneys because of pressure differences, increasing the risk of kidney damage and impaired function.

The growth of the prostate gland is usually benign and is thought to be caused by an accumulation of the male sex hormone testosterone in the prostate, where it is converted to a potent chemical called dihydrotestosterone (DHT). It is DHT that causes the enlargement.

Regular rectal examinations are important because a doctor can detect from the texture of the enlarged gland whether there is a likelihood of cancer and early diagnosis is vital.

4

TREATMENT
Orthodox treatment is usually surgery. Partial removal of the prostate gland means that any remnants will still retain the tendency to grow, however, so the treatment may need to be repeated in time, while complete removal can lead to impotence or erectile difficulties.

■ Saw palmetto can actively combat enlargement by reducing production of DHT. Mix two parts each of saw palmetto and Siberian ginseng tinctures with one part white deadnettle and take 5 ml three times a day. Saw palmetto is also available in capsules.

■ Urinary antiseptics will help deal with any infection caused by the residual urine. If there are signs of urethritis or cystitis, drink a cup of infusion containing equal amounts of corn silk, white deadnettle and buchu three times a day; add one teaspoon of horsetail juice to each cup.

■ Studies carried out in Germany suggest that stinging nettle extracts may also combat prostate enlargement, so drink regular cups of infusion or take ready-made tablets.

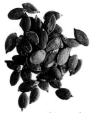

pumpkin seeds

■ Zinc has a beneficial effect on the prostate gland and will also help to reduce the overall size of the gland – take 15 mg daily or eat plenty of pumpkin seeds, which are a good natural source.

■ Recent studies have also demonstrated that tomatoes contain a chemical which can also help to combat prostate enlargement – eat a portion of tomatoes every day, either in salads or cooked dishes, or drink a glass of tomato juice at breakfast.

SAW PALMETTO

As well as being an important Native American medicinal herb, saw palmetto berries were a favourite foodstuff while the wood and twigs were used to make brooms, hats and baskets. The root was variously used for treating dysentery, kidney disorders, sore eyes and high blood pressure by different Indian tribes. Settlers noticed that animals feeding on the berries grew sleek and fat, so they turned them into tonic wines for domestic use.

In recent years researchers have demonstrated that saw palmetto can both prevent benign prostate enlargement, by preventing the conversion of the male hormone testosterone into dihydrotestosterone, and help to cure it, since the berries also encourage breakdown of any DHT that may have formed.

4

PROSTATITIS

Inflammation of the prostate gland is often due to bacterial infection, with symptoms very similar to urethritis (see p.88). There may be pain in the crotch and lower back, discomfort on passing urine and possibly also a mild fever and raised temperature.

REMEDIES

■ Make an infusion containing equal amounts of white deadnettle, buchu and golden rod and add one tablespoon of horsetail juice to each cup; drink three cups daily.

■ In addition echinacea will help to combat the infection and protect the kidneys – take up to 600 mg in capsules of 5 ml of tincture, three times daily.

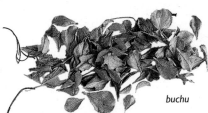

buchu

URINARY TRACT PROBLEMS

Urinary tract infections ascend through the urethra – the narrow tube that takes urine from the bladder to outside the body. The urethra is very much shorter in women than in men, so while women usually suffer from cystitis (inflammation of the bladder), infections are less likely to reach the male bladder and men tend to suffer from urethritis (inflammation of the urethra) instead.

CYSTITIS AND URETHRITIS

Symptoms can include a burning sensation on passing urine, a frequent need to do so, dull aches in the lower abdomen, and possibly blood in the urine. Some types of urethritis can be associated with sexually transmitted diseases and in the UK must be referred to specialist clinics.

yarrow

cornsilk

buchu

- Make a tea containing equal amounts of buchu, yarrow and cornsilk (one teaspoon of the mix per cup) and drink a cup every three or four hours while symptoms persist.

- If there is blood in the urine, then add an equal amount of shepherd's purse to the above mix.

- Useful alternative herbs for teas include bearberry, couchgrass, celery seed and agrimony.

- Cranberry juice has proved very effective in clinical trials; drink at least six glasses of the unsweetened juice daily.

4

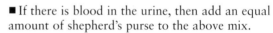

YARROW

Yarrow is a common meadow plant which is astringent, bitter, anti-inflammatory, diaphoretic, diuretic and styptic. It is useful for cystitis and urethritis, especially when there is blood in the urine. It relaxes the peripheral blood vessels, so can help to reduce high blood pressure and it is also cooling in fevers.

Yarrow flowers – like those of chamomile – contain anti-allergenic compounds which are activated by hot water and so are produced only in infusions, the essential oil and in steam inhalations. These can be useful for easing the symptoms of asthma and hay fever.

Yarrow should be avoided in pregnancy as it is a uterine stimulant. The fresh herb can sometimes cause contact dermatitis.

HERBS FOR CHILDREN

Sick children are a major source of worry to their parents – not only due to concerns about the illness but because their symptoms can vary so dramatically and suddenly. Soaring temperatures can occur within minutes while a child's normal pulse and breathing rates are much faster than adults anyway so the fever symptoms appear to be worse than they are.

Fever can subside as suddenly as it started, and many parents have summoned urgent medical help only to have an apparently well toddler running around by the time the doctor arrives. See the pointers on p.100 for when to summon medical help.

Herbs can prove gentle and soothing for even quite young children – but little ones may require persuasion to swallow their bitter tasting remedies. Drops of tincture on a spoonful of honey are often the easiest way to administer the remedy.

BABIES AND TODDLERS

Babies and toddlers often respond well to herbal remedies. Many babies will happily take very weak herbal infusions from a bottle in their first months, and once the practice has been established they're likely to be quite happy about swallowing herbal remedies as they grow older without any fuss or complaints about the taste.

COLIC

Poor positioning on the nipple or teat, so that the baby swallows air as it sucks, is probably the commonest cause of colic. The baby's crying at the resulting pain increases the mother's tension and compounds the problem.

If breast-feeding, drinking a relaxing cup of chamomile or vervain tea in between feeds will help. Irritant foods, such as hot spices, cow's milk or wheat, are easily transferred to breast milk. If there is a history of allergies in the family, the breast-feeding mother should take special care with her own diet.

RELIEF AND RELAXATION

■ Catmint is ideal to soothe gut spasm and encourage sleep. Make an infusion using one teaspoon of dried catmint to 500 ml of water, and give the baby one to two tablespoons of the warm infusion before meals. The surplus can be stored in a refrigerator for up to 48 hours and reheated before use.

■ Dill, fennel and caraway can be made into teas for the baby in the same way or be taken by the mother before feeds.

■ Soak a compress in an infusion of chamomile flowers and apply to the baby's abdomen, or give one to two drops of homoeopathic chamomile (Chamomilla 3X) every 15 minutes.

■ Try traditional Chinese baby massage: stroke the baby's lower spine from the lumbar region to the coccyx up to 200 times in one direction. For diarrhoea, stroke from coccyx to lumbar area; for constipation, stroke in the opposite direction.

5

SLEEPLESSNESS

There can often be a simple explanation for sleeplessness in a baby – she may be too hot, too cold, hungry or suffering from colic, or she may just want the company of her parents. Always make sure the baby is comfortable, feels safe and secure, and has plenty of cuddles before bed. Moving the cot to the parental bedroom can help.

CALM BEFORE BEDTIME

■ Add a cup of chamomile infusion or two drops of chamomile oil to the baby's bath water each night to help her relax – make sure oils are well dispersed in the water.

■ Gentle Chinese massage can calm small babies: stroke the forearms slowly in one direction for 100 strokes, using a little dilute chamomile oil (one drop in 20 ml sweet almond oil) on your finger.

■ Breast-feeding mothers could drink a cup of chamomile, Californian poppy, lemon balm or lime blossom tea before the bedtime feed, or if the baby will take a bottle, offer an infusion (one teaspoon of herb to 500 ml water in tablespoon doses) of the same herbs about 20 minutes before bedtime.

TEETHING

The teeth start to appear from around four months, though some babies cut their first teeth earlier. It can be painful; massaging the baby's gums with a herbal mixture can bring relief.

TREATMENT

■ Mix two drops each of chamomile, sage and rosemary oils in two tablespoons of sunflower or almond oil; store in a clean bottle. Smear a little oil on your finger and gently rub onto the baby's gums. Repeat three or four times a day as necessary.

■ Try giving the baby the herbal teas suggestions given under Sleeplessness, above, to calm her, or give homoeopathic Chamomilla 3X pillules or drops as required.

■ A traditional Chinese remedy to ease teething pains is to put one drop of clove oil in a teaspoon of almond oil and use to gently massage the baby's lower back.

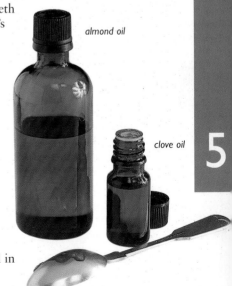

almond oil

clove oil

5

MARIGOLD

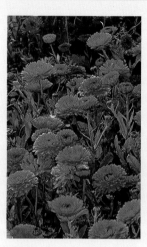

One of our most popular herbs, marigold is widely available in commercial creams and ointments although it is just as valuable as an internal remedy. The plant is astringent, antiseptic, anti-fungal, and anti-inflammatory and can help to regulate the menstrual cycle and stimulate bile production to improve the digestion.

The cream is usually sold under marigold's botanical name of *Calendula*, and is a valuable household standby for skin rashes and sores, cuts, grazes, vaginal thrush, eczema, sore nipples in breast-feeding and numerous other problems.

Marigold cream is safe and soothing for a number of childhood problems including nappy rash and eczema as well as a useful first-aid remedy for accidental knocks and scrapes.

NAPPY RASH

This painful red rash is extremely common, and while it can be related to infrequent nappy changes or inefficient cleansing, it can also suggest digestive problems and yeast infections. Breast-feeding mothers should examine their own diets for any excess of refined carbohydrates, alcohol, processed foods or dairy products which may encourage fungal growths.

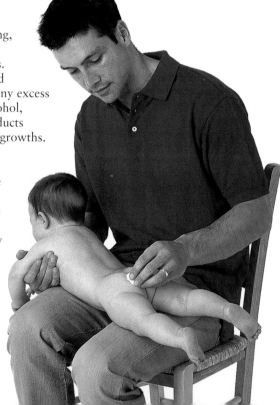

SOOTHING THE RASH
■ Use an infusion of heartsease to wash the affected area (add one drop of tea tree oil if there is any sign of infection). Make sure the baby is completely dry – leave the nappy off as long as possible when changing.

■ Apply either comfrey or marigold oils or ointments. Ointments are better than creams in this case as they form a protective waterproof coating.

5

CRADLE CAP

A type of scaly dermatitis which affects the scalps of new babies, cradle cap is an unsightly condition, however, it is neither serious nor contagious. In fact it is more of a worry for the new mother than an irritant for the baby.

Heartsease is the traditional remedy of choice: either bathe the scalp with an infusion of heartsease three or four times a day, taking great care with new babies where the fontanelles (the soft spots between the skull bones) have yet to close completely, or apply infused heartsease oil or cream. Infused marigold oil is also suitable – rub either oil into the baby's scalp several times a day.

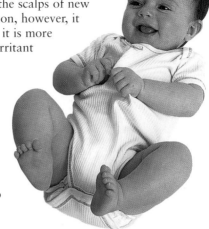

BEDWETTING

Most toddlers wet the bed occasionally until the bladder matures. For a few, however, it can remain a problem well into school age. Bedwetting may be a habit, or it may be related to minor sub-clinical urinary infections, dietary imbalance, problems with the urinary tract or emotional upsets. It is important to find the cause. If there may be a physical problem, medical help is needed.

REMEDIES

■ Limiting fluids in the two or three hours before bedtime is a common stratagem, though it is not always successful.

■ In some cases a contrived ritual can help – drops of herbal tincture on the tongue before bedtime add an aura of magic to the remedy and enhance any potential placebo affect as well.

■ Try drops of cornsilk or St. John's wort tinctures, or else use an infusion containing equal amounts of these herbs with a little honey and give half a cup three times a day. Unpasteurised honey should not be given to children under 2.

■ A teaspoon of horsetail juice given three times a day will help to strengthen the urinary system.

5

INFECTIONS

The familiar infections of childhood are usually fairly minor and respond well to simple home remedies – but complications can occur and sometimes (as in measles) professional help is essential. Most of the problems are caused by viruses so antibiotics will have no effect and herbal remedies to strengthen the immune system can be ideal. For general immune tonics, see Infections, p.42.

CHICKEN POX

Also known as varicella, this contagious viral disease typically starts with red spots on the chest and back, gradually spreading to the rest of the body, scalp and face. The irritant spots develop into blisters, then scabs. Scratching or damaging these can lead to scars, so it is important to take great care when bathing infected children. Other symptoms include a slightly raised temperature (39–40°C/102–104°F), sore throat and nasal congestion.

GETTING BACK TO HEALTH

Treatment usually involves strengthening the immune system and easing the symptoms while the body attacks the virus.

■ A lotion made from equal amounts of chickweed infusion, borage juice and distilled witch hazel can be used on the irritant skin rash – apply with a cotton wool swab every one to two hours or as required.

■ Give the child echinacea capsules tincture (dose dependent on age) three times daily to stimulate the immune system.

■ Soothe any irritability by giving infusions of skullcap, wood betony or chamomile as required.

■ During the feverish stage of the disease apply cool compresses or sponges soaked in marigold, borage or basil infusions. Keeping the patient cool will also reduce the irritation of the skin rash.

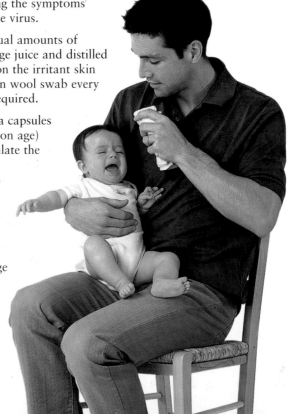

5

MEASLES
· ·

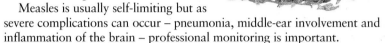

Measles is a highly contagious viral disease. Symptoms include catarrh, watery bloodshot eyes and increased sensitivity to light, fever (up to 40°C/104°F), a harsh dry cough and a blotchy rash usually starting behind the ears. Incubation is up to two weeks.

Measles is usually self-limiting but as severe complications can occur – pneumonia, middle-ear involvement and inflammation of the brain – professional monitoring is important.

RELIEVING SYMPTOMS
■ Ease the cough with an infusion of equal amounts of marshmallow leaf, hyssop and ribwort plantain (half a cup up to four times daily; smaller doses for younger children). Regular doses of echinacea will support the immune system.

■ Eyebaths made from a well-strained infusion of eyebright, self-heal or elder flowers will also help – there is a risk of permanent sight damage in measles, so seek medical help if there is any inflammation or the condition worsens.

■ Sponge a feverish child with a marigold or basil infusion and give calming herbal teas to make her more comfortable.

MUMPS
· ·

This viral infection involves inflammation of the salivary glands with painful swelling in front of the ears. Typical symptoms include general malaise and headache followed by a fever (up to 40°C/104°F) and swelling in the neck. With children the condition is usually mild and suitable for home treatment but adult sufferers should seek professional help as there is a risk of sterility.

TREATMENT
■ Take echinacea or garlic regularly to boost the immune system.

■ Gargle with an antiseptic infusion made from equal amounts of thyme and sage (two teaspoons of the mix to a cup of water). Strain and cool before gargling.

■ Fresh cleavers juice will help with the glandular involvement (one tablespoon in water every three to four hours). Apply infused St. John's wort oil or a hot compress soaked in St. John's wort infusion to the neck and face.

■ In adults chaste-tree or pasque flower can be helpful if the testicles or ovaries are involved (40 drops of either tincture two to three times daily).

■ Drink plenty of yarrow, angelica and marigold tea (one to two teaspoons of the mix per cup for adults, less for children).

5

INFESTATIONS

Parasites such as head lice, threadworms and pinworms are common and spread easily – they are not necessarily a sign of poor hygiene. Simple herbal treatments and preventative measures to stop the infestation from spreading are usually all that is needed.

NITS AND HEAD LICE

Lice infect the scalp and lay their eggs (nits) firmly attached to the roots of the hair, where they can be difficult to remove. They are commonplace in school outbreaks – suspect infection if children persistently scratch their heads. There are effective herbal alternatives to the usual powerful insecticidal shampoos.

HERBAL HELP
■ Mix equal amounts of tea tree, thyme and lemon essential oils; add ten drops to 500 ml of warm water and use as a final rinse after shampooing. Repeat every few days until the infection clears.

■ Use the same oils, in 10 ml of sweet almond oil, to soak a fine-toothed comb and comb the child's hair thoroughly. Repeat two to three times a day until the infection clears.

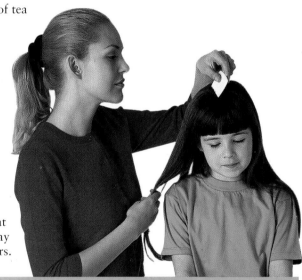

LEMON BALM

Lemon balm is closely associated with bees and the healing power of honey, and was regarded by the ancient Greeks as something of a cure-all.

It is mostly used as a carminative and sedative, although the plant is also valuable as a diaphoretic to lower body temperature and is anti-viral so can be especially useful for familiar childhood infections. It is a gentle herb – ideal for treating nervous tummy upsets in children but also potent enough to help with conditions such as depression, anxiety and tension headaches.

Externally, lemon balm creams can be used on insect bites, sores and slow-healing wounds. The essential oil is used in aromatherapy for nervous problems and is also valuable, well-diluted in sprays, for keeping insects away.

5

CHILDHOOD DOSES

Children's dosages vary depending on the age or body weight of the child. Seek professional advice before giving any herb internally to very young babies apart from the suggestions given in this chapter for bottle-fed infusions. The dosages can be gradually increased from one age range to the next.

Age	Dosage
6–12 months	$\frac{1}{10}$ adult dose
1–2 years	$\frac{1}{5}$ adult dose
3–4 years	$\frac{1}{4}$ adult dose
6–7 years	$\frac{1}{3}$ adult dose
9–10 years	$\frac{1}{2}$ adult dose
Puberty	Full adult dose

WORMS

Threadworms and pinworms are common infestations in children. They are also highly contagious and can easily spread to other family members (including adults) so scrupulous hygiene is essential. Ensure that everyone washes their hands thoroughly after visiting the lavatory and try to keep separate towels for each person. Female worms lay eggs at the anus at night so examine the child's bottom before bedtime and remove worms with tweezers.

TREATMENT
■ Herbs can be effective at killing the worms. Put ten drops each of wormwood and fennel tinctures in a glass of either cabbage or carrot juice. Stir well and give the child a glassful to drink each morning before breakfast for four days. Repeat the treatment two weeks later (treatment needs to be repeated to mirror the worm's life cycle).

■ Garlic will also clear worms so use plenty in your cooking or give children garlic pearles on a regular basis as a preventative if you feel they are at risk from re-infection. For children who cannot swallow capsules, mix the contents of a pearle or half a finely chopped clove with a teaspoon of honey.

5

ALLERGIES

Pollution, excess use of antibiotics and food additives have all been blamed for the rapid growth in childhood allergies in recent years. Identifying the allergen is essential but eliminating it is not always easy – especially since the child may become addicted to the cause of the problem.

HYPERACTIVITY

All children are active, but hyperactivity is in a different league. Symptoms can include sleeplessness, poor attention span, aggression and learning difficulties. Some aspects of hyperactivity have been linked with forms of dyslexia. Food intolerance or pollution may be to blame, or there may be emotional difficulties.

■ Calming herbal teas can help. Make an infusion containing equal amounts of wood betony, self-heal and borage; give half to one cup up to three times a day.

■ Evening primrose or borage oil as a dietary supplement can help (250–500 mg daily). Look for ready-made capsules which also contain a little thyme oil – this has been shown to help in dyslexia and cases of poor concentration.

■ If environmental pollution is contributing to the problem, give the child a daily kelp supplement which can help cleanse heavy metals from the system.

CHILDHOOD ECZEMA

Allergic eczema (see also p.45) generally starts at weaning – cows' milk is usually suspected. Irritant rashes may cover the child's entire body. Orthodox treatment usually depends on steroidal creams – these should be used as sparingly as possible. Keeping the child cool, especially at night, can reduce the irritation.

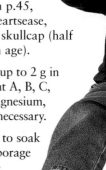

■ As well as the remedies suggested on p.45, try an infusion of equal amounts of heartsease, red clover flowers, stinging nettle and skullcap (half to one teaspoon per cup depending on age).

■ Evening primrose oil may help – give up to 2 g in capsules daily. Ensure there are sufficient A, B, C, and E vitamins in the diet as well as magnesium, zinc and calcium – give supplements if necessary.

■ Borage juice can soothe rashes (use it to soak a compress or apply as a lotion). Add borage to your infusion mixture to combat the effects of steroid creams if they have been used for any length of time.

5

GLUE EAR

Glue ear, or secretory otitis media, is a common childhood problem which some researchers now associate with milk allergies. Symptoms include recurrent ear infections, progressive hearing loss, and copious sticky secretions from the ear. Orthodox treatment usually involves surgical insertion of grommets in the eardrums to relieve the fluid build-up.

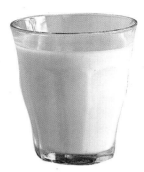

TREATMENT

■ Make an infusion from equal amounts of golden rod, ginkgo leaves, ribwort plantain and St. John's wort and give one tablespoon to a cup (depending on age) up to three times daily.

■ Use mullein oil or garlic oil as ear drops (as long as there is no perforation of the ear drum and grommets have not been inserted).

■ Try excluding all cow's milk and milk products from the diet for at least three weeks.

ELDER

The elder tree was traditionally regarded as a complete medicine chest, with all parts of the plant used in some way. The leaves were made into a "green ointment" for sprains and strains, the bark used as a strong purgative for constipation, the berries, rich in vitamin C, to combat colds and infections, and the flowers as an anti-catarrhal and anti-inflammatory.

Today our use is largely limited to the flowers, which are also made into commercial hand creams and cordials. Elder flowers also strengthen the mucous membranes and help increase resistance to allergens.

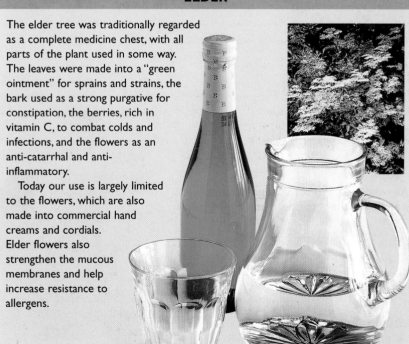

5

STOMACH UPSETS

While children can suffer the same sorts of digestive problems as adults (see pp.24–27 and 52–55) they are also more susceptible to non-specific "bilious attacks" and travel sickness.

GASTRIC UPSETS

Many children suffer from regular "bilious attacks" or gastric disturbances – usually with nausea, vomiting, diarrhoea, general malaise, headache or tummy pains. Always seek professional advice for any gastric upsets in children lasting for more than 12 hours.

■ Make an infusion containing equal amounts of agrimony and wood betony and give two tablespoons to one cup up to three times a day.

■ Use a cool compress soaked in lavender infusion to soothe headaches or a warm compress soaked in cramp bark decoction for abdominal pains.

■ Ensure adequate fluid intake to prevent dehydration if the child suffers from protracted diarrhoea or vomiting.

TRAVEL SICKNESS

Motion sickness may be caused by a stuffy atmosphere, diesel fumes or restricted vision upsetting the balance of the inner ear.

■ Ginger is a good preventative. Give the child ginger tablets or capsules if she can swallow them, or use drops of dilute tincture on the tongue, about half an hour before travelling – repeat if necessary during the journey. Ginger biscuits, crystallized ginger sweets or ginger beer can be almost as effective. Galangal can be used in the same way.

■ Alternatively, use chamomile, lemon balm or meadowsweet infusion or tinctures before and during the journey.

WHEN TO SEEK HELP FOR SICK CHILDREN	
If your child's symptoms include any of the following, seek professional help as a matter of urgency:	■ Severe diarrhoea or vomiting.
	■ Milder diarrhoea which continues for more than 12 hours.
■ Convulsions or fits.	■ The child complains of neck stiffness accompanied by signs of fever, headache or a rash.
■ Breathing problems or unusual drowsiness and lethargy.	
■ An unusual, high-pitched cry in babies and toddlers.	■ Temperature above 39°C/102°F for more than a couple of hours.

5

HERBS TO KEEP YOU HEALTHY

Herbs are not only helpful when we're ill, they can also play an important role in keeping us healthy. We now know that many herbs have significant therapeutic properties to combat the effects of ageing and pollution or strengthen the immune system.

Sage and rosemary, traditionally associated with longevity, contain antioxidants to counter free radicals, while traditional energy tonics like ginseng are rich in hormone-like compounds that have a significant effect on human metabolism. Other herbs can help us relax more effectively or stimulate the immune system or vital energy. But while herbs, like healthy foods, can strengthen the system and help it cope with life's daily demands, they are no substitute for a healthy lifestyle with plenty of relaxation and invigorating exercise, a well-balanced outlook on life, and a degree of contentment.

IMMUNE STIMULANTS

Many herbs were traditionally used to combat infections, and modern research has shown that these plants are not only anti-bacterial and anti-fungal, but some are also anti-viral – so they really can help with colds and influenza. Others stimulate the immune system, so helping it to overcome invading pathogens.

ECHINACEA

Also known as purple cone flower, echinacea was used by Native Americans healers for an impressive array of ailments, from snake bite to toothache. Three closely related species are used for a broad spectrum of infections – *E. pallida*, *E. purpurea* and *E. angustifolia*. Although the root has been most commonly used, recent research has demonstrated that the aerial parts of *E. purpurea* are just as effective. The seeds are readily available from garden centres for growing plants at home.

echinacea capsules

As well as treating colds, echinacea is used for kidney and urinary infections and septicaemia and it is also made into creams for external use on cuts, grazes and skin infections.

Although many herbalists prefer to use echinacea in relatively high doses for treating acute infections (up to 800 mg in capsules or 10 ml in tincture per dose), others regard a low regular dose (one 200 mg capsule daily) as a useful preventive, especially for school-age children.

ASTRAGALUS

Known in China as *huang qi* or milk vetch in English, astragalus is one of the most important tonic herbs used in traditional Chinese medicine. It acts as a stimulant for the immune system and has a tonic effect on lungs, stomach and kidney. Astragalus is diuretic, strengthens the body's vital energy (*qi*), encourages tissue regeneration, reduces swellings and clears pus.

The root is widely used in traditional remedies for palpitations, debility, kidney disease, chest problems and slow-to-heal boils and sores. Studies also suggest that astragalus can help strengthen the immune system in cancer patients.

In China, astragalus is regarded as a more suitable general energy tonic for younger people than ginseng, although its strong immune-strengthening effects make it valuable for recurrent infections, slow-healing wounds and general debility. The root is sold in Chinese herb shops in slices and a typical dose is 9–15 g in decoction.

6

astragalus slices

SHIITAKE MUSHROOMS

Now easily found on supermarket shelves, shiitake mushrooms are anti-viral and anti-tumour, lower cholesterol levels, act as a liver tonic and stimulate the immune system. Extracts of the mushroom have been used in Japan with patients undergoing chemotherapy and studies have shown that they can reduce the growth rate of liver tumours. Shiitake extracts have also been used in the treatment of AIDS.

The mushroom has been used in Chinese medicine for at least 2,000 years, although shiitake is actually the Japanese name – the Chinese call it *xiang gu*.

In traditional Chinese medicine the typical dose is 6–16 g dried mushroom or 90 g fresh, taken in a soup up to three times a day. This dose is quite high by Western standards and might lead to gastric upsets, so opt instead for the commercial extracts which concentrate the active ingredients, or else use more conventional amounts of the mushrooms in cooking.

MAKING DECOCTIONS

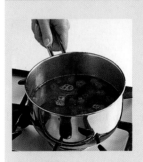

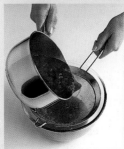

Tough materials such as roots, berries and barks need to be made into decoctions to extract the active ingredients. The traditional Western dose is 30 g of dried root to 750 ml of water, simmered until the volume has reduced by about a third, then strained and used in three wine-glass doses a day.

Chinese herbs, such as astragalus, are generally used in higher doses, but start with these proportions and increase the dose only if you do not suffer from digestive upsets or other side effects.

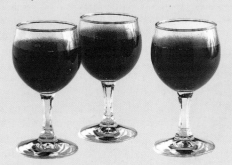

6

ENERGY TONICS

Herbal traditions put great emphasis on the body's inner vital energy. As late as the 19th century, Western practitioners still used remedies to strengthen the "vital force" while the Eastern concepts of *qi* and *prana* have become very familiar to modern Westerners. Many herbs have been used to strengthen this inner energy – from traditional European plants to exotic newcomers like guarana and Peruvian cat's claw which are now easily available from health food stores.

GINSENG

Ginseng has been used in China for more than 5,000 years to strengthen *qi* – the body's vital energy. It is rich in steroidal compounds which are very similar to human sex hormones – hence its reputation as an aphrodisiac. It is also a good all-round tonic helping the body adapt to stressful situations, stimulating the immune system and energy levels and having a specific tonic action on the lungs and spleen.

In Chinese tradition, ginseng is recommended only for the over-40s. It is best taken as a revitalizing tonic for up to a month in late autumn to strengthen the system for the winter, although many devotees take the herb all year round. The usual dose is 600 mg in capsules daily or it can be made into decoctions and tonic wines.

High doses of ginseng are best avoided in pregnancy although it may be taken for short periods then. Other herbal stimulants, such as caffeine-containing drinks should be avoided while taking ginseng.

DAMIANA

Damiana is one of the many tonic and aphrodisiac herbs that originate from Central and South America. The plant is a strongly aromatic shrub which acts as a tonic for the nervous system and is antidepressant, stimulating for the digestion and urinary system, an energy-giving tonic and an aphrodisiac. The leaves and stems are used.

Damiana is a useful tonic in convalescence and general debility and stimulates the appetite. Helpful for menstrual problems, it can be used to treat loss of libido, impotence and prostate problems. Aromatherapists use the essential oil in tonic and uplifting massage.

6

ELECAMPANE

A herb with a long history, elecampane was regarded as something of a cure-all by the Romans, who used it to treat a wide range of conditions including menstrual problems, digestive upsets, dropsy and sciatica. The Anglo-Saxons believed it to be a magical herb, proof against elf-shot and the evil eye, and also used it as a cure for skin disease and leprosy.

Today we know elecampane as an important expectorant and lung tonic used in cough and catarrh remedies. The root can be used to shift phlegm and is particularly useful in clearing coughs and congestion in children. It also contains inulin, a polysaccharaide which has been used as a sugar substitute in diabetes.

Elecampane is also diaphoretic (causing sweat) and diuretic and has anti-bacterial and anti-fungal properties. Chinese research has shown that it stimulates the nervous and digestive systems.

As a tonic, elecampane is ideally suited to combating the depression, lingering coughs and debility that can follow a bout of flu, and also in asthmatic and bronchitic conditions. Although the root is the part used in Western herbalism, the Chinese prefer the flowers of a related species, *Inula japonica*.

CHINESE ANGELICA (DANG GUI)

Dang gui is one of China's most important tonic herbs. It has been used for a range of gynaecological problems for at least 2,000 years and is said to "nourish the blood" so can be helpful for anaemia, menstrual problems including period pain, or as a tonic after childbirth.

This versatile herb is a painkiller, blood tonic and circulatory stimulant, a liver stimulant, clearing stagnation of toxins and energy, and has some anti-bacterial action, while its mild laxative action and energizing properties make it helpful for constipation in the elderly. It is very widely used in traditional Chinese medicine and has also become familiar in Western herbalism. *Dang gui* – also called in the west *tang kwai* or *dong quai* – is also widely used in general purpose tonic preparations targeted at women. Ready-made products are increasingly popular and widely available.

6

MIND AND SPIRIT TONICS

Although Western medicine tends to focus on physical remedies, an holistic approach also takes into account emotional and spiritual aspects, and herbs have a long tradition in these areas. As well as the remedies earlier suggested for the emotions (p.60–63) try some of these.

GOTU KOLA

Also known as Indian pennywort, gotu kola is one of the most important Ayurvedic tonic herbs. It has long been used as a rejuvenating remedy, to counter the problems of old age and improve memory. In the East is it also used to treat leprosy. It can be helpful for many skin conditions and will clear scar tissue.

Although gotu kola has been used for conditions as diverse as malaria and venereal disease, it tends to be regarded as a nervine and tonic in the West. It is included in many over-the-counter tonic mixtures, or can be taken in infusion.

BASIL

Widely used in Europe as a culinary herb, basil is regarded in India as a potent tonic, and is one of the most sacred plants in the Ayurvedic repertoire. It is described as opening the heart and mind, increasing our energy for love and devotion and improving faith, compassion and clarity. Basil is carminative, warming, antispasmodic, anti-bacterial and analgesic and has been used to clear intestinal parasites and improve digestion. The oil is used as a nerve tonic, antidepressant and digestive remedy but should be avoided in pregnancy.

VERVAIN

Once known as "herb of grace", vervain was regarded as sacred to the god Jove by the Romans. The herb was used in divination by the druids and given to babies to help them learn more quickly. Today it is used as relaxing nervine and liver tonic. It is bitter, stimulating for the digestion, ideal as a tonic in convalescence and debility, sedating and calming, and helpful for neuralgia and migraine.

Mystics sometimes claim that vervain can heal holes in the human aura, so strengthening the energy forces surrounding us. It should be avoided in pregnancy but can be taken in labour to stimulate contractions.

REISHI MUSHROOM

Reishi is a type of bracket fungus known as *ling zhi* in China, and was one of the most important herbs of the ancient Chinese Taoists. The Taoists followed a way of life which concentrated on achieving prosperity, longevity and even immortality through virtue – which in this context meant conformity to nature both within the individual and beyond. To the Taoists, reishi was one of the herbs that could strengthen the adherence to virtue which they believed to be essential for a long life and good fortune.

The herb is a nervine and heart tonic and has anti-bacterial, anti-allergenic and anti-tussive (anti-cough) properties. It is a potent immune stimulant and anti-tumour herb, and has been used in the treatment of chronic fatigue syndrome (ME) and AIDS. It can also be used for high blood pressure and chronic asthma. As a tonic for the mind, it seems to give courage to change our lives: to resolve and follow a determined cause of action or better way of life.

MAKING TONIC WINES

A daily glass of tonic wine is a delightful way to take herbal remedies. Ideally use an earthenware vinegar vat, although a large rumpot or glass jar are also suitable. Fill the vat with the chosen tonic herb – ideally using a root remedy like ginger, liquorice or *dang gui* rather than leafy parts – and cover with a good quality red wine (preferably organic). Leave the mix for at least two weeks before drawing the liquid off in a daily sherry glass dose. Keep the herb covered with more red wine to prevent it from going mouldy. The wine will continue to extract active constituents from the roots for several months before you need to replace the herb.

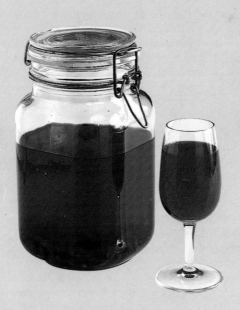

6

HERBAL TEAS

Herbal "teas" can be made either by infusing the aerial parts of the herb (see p.51) or by decocting the tougher roots or berries (p.103). You can make a combined infusion/decoction by first decocting the tough plant components and then pouring the mix over the dried aerial parts and infusing for ten minutes. While herbal teas are frequently recommended for specific ailments, they also make refreshing or relaxing brews for everyday drinking.

RELAXING TEAS

Experiment with combinations of any of the relaxing herbs such as wood betony, chamomile, skullcap, vervain, lemon balm, St. John's wort or lavender, or take them separately if you prefer. Try mixing equal amounts of lemon balm, chamomile flowers and lime flowers. Store the mixture in a glass or ceramic jar, use one teaspoon per cup and infuse for five to ten minutes before drinking.

There are also plenty of herbs to add to night-time brews to ensure a good night's sleep. As well as the relaxing plants mentioned above, try those listed on pp.67–68. A traditional Welsh night-time drink was made by mixing equal amounts of red clover flowers, hops and wild lettuce (one to two teaspoons per cup of infusion). The great French herbalist Maurice Mességué suggested combining equal amounts of wild lettuce, hawthorn flowers, melilot and red corn poppies (you could use Californian poppies instead). Use two teaspoons of the mixture per mug, infuse for five to ten minutes and drink the hot brew 20–30 minutes before bedtime.

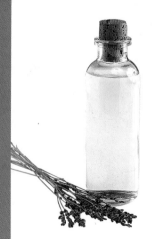

LAVENDER

The name of this useful and fragrant herb comes from the Latin verb *lavare* – to wash. Lavender is regarded as an antiseptic and cleansing remedy, and has been widely used in perfumes and toiletries for centuries.

The herb is also antispasmodic and carminative so it is a useful treatment for digestive problems. It is uplifting and antidepressant and is helpful for tension and emotional upsets, as well as a cooling remedy for migraines and headaches.

Lavender is also traditionally used for treating headaches which are eased by an ice-pack, while rosemary is better for those head pains that respond to a hot compress.

Herbal medicine tends to use the oil, collected by steam distillation – its antiseptic properties make it an essential addition to the first-aid box. The flowers, while less potent, are delicious in home-made teas.

CHAMOMILE

Chamomile flowers make a popular tisane, although commercial tea bags all too often lack the pungency of the fresh herb. Two species are used medicinally – Roman chamomile (*Chamaemelum nobile*) and German chamomile (*Matricaria recutita*). Their properties are very similar. Two or three fresh flowers are all you need add to a cup of boiling water to make a delicious night time drink which will help relieve insomnia, anxiety and stress. A cup of chamomile tea can also be added to baby's bath water or (if well diluted) bottle-feeds to ease both sleeplessness and the traumas of teething.

Chamomile is carminative and soothing for the minor digestive upsets – as an anti-inflammatory and antispasmodic it will also help to relieve symptoms of chronic conditions, such as irritable bowel syndrome.

Chamomile creams and ointments are ideal for a wide range of skin irritations including insect bites and eczema and they will also help to relieve anal and vaginal itching. The infusion makes a good steam inhalation for hay fever and to combat minor asthmatic problems. The same mix will also soothe congestive cararrh and bronchitis.

SKULLCAP

Virginian skullcap was introduced into Europe in the 18th century as a treatment for rabies – hence its alternative name of mad dog herb. Although it was traditionally used by the Native Americans as a remedy for menstrual problems, it is now valued more as an effective sedative and nervine, and can be used to treat nervous exhuastion and premenstrual tension.

Skullcap is cooling, antibacterial, styptic, will reduce fevers, lower blood pressure and cholesterol levels, and stimulates digestion. It has a pleasant flavour and is a useful addition to relaxing teas. The European variety of skullcap (*Scutellaria galericulata*) has similar properties. The Chinese use another variety, *S. baicalensis* (*huang qin*).

STORING HERBS

When buying dried herbs, choose suppliers that store the herbs in dark glass jars kept out of the light – direct sunlight makes herbs deteriorate more quickly – and always buy herbs that look fresh and well-coloured rather than drab and dusty.

If you dry your own herbs, hang the stems in small bunches away from direct light and with a good circulation of air. Herbs collected on a dry day in summer should be dry enough to crush and store within four or five days. If you are drying seeds or flowers, tie a paper bag loosely over the stems to catch any seeds or florets that fall.

It is always easiest to mix your dried herbs in bulk for tea making. Use 25–50 g (1–2 oz) of each herb in your combination and mix them together well in a large bowl. Spoon the mix into a clean dark glass or ceramic jar with an air-tight lid, and store in a cool place away from direct sunlight.

6

STIMULATING TEAS

Our most obviously stimulating beverages are ordinary Indian tea and coffee –
both perfectly good herbal remedies (tea is highly astringent, so good for
diarrhoea) although their caffeine-like alkaloids give a rather artificial
stimulation compared with the herbal energy tonics described on pp.104–105.

   Well-chosen combinations of herbs can also deliver the stimulation needed
first thing in the morning, or to keep us alert when working hard. Traditional
herbal morning teas usually combine a mixture of digestive remedies to start
the day and astringents and tonic plants to help stimulate the system.

■ One pleasant-tasting combination, based on a traditional Austrian drink,
combines equal quantities of peppermint, hibiscus flowers, strawberry leaves,
raspberry leaves, marigold petals, chamomile flowers and cornflowers. Use
one to two teaspoons of the mixture per cup; infuse for five to ten minutes.
The mixture makes a cheerful and colourful start to the day.

■ Another uplifting mix, based on an original recipe by the French herbalist
Maurice Mességué, is made by combining equal amounts of chamomile
flowers, wood betony, peppermint, lime flowers and lavender. Use one to two
teaspoons of the mixture per cup, infused for five to ten minutes.

■ A good stimulating mix for when you are studying or working hard is made
by combining equal amounts of rosemary, gotu kola and sage. Use one
teaspoon of the mixture per cup, infused for five minutes.

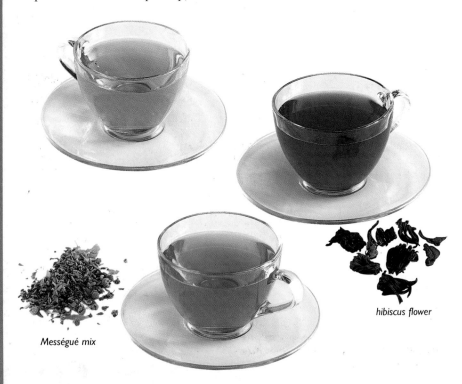

hibiscus flower

Mességué mix

6

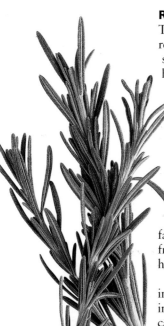

ROSEMARY

This Mediterranean shrub was traditionally regarded as a very warming plant that was both stimulating and uplifting. The Elizabethan herbalist, John Gerard, suggested that it "comforteth the harte and maketh it merrie" while earlier writers believed that simply smelling the plant frequently would keep you young and vigorous.

The tonic action of rosemary is largely due to a stimulating substance called borneol. The herb is also strongly antioxidant to combat cell decay and has a practical and invigorating effect on our bodies.

It makes a pleasant tea for temporary fatigue and over-work and, as it is evergreen, the fresh leaves are available all year round once you have established a bush in your garden.

As well as being generally stimulating, rosemary infusion is helpful for headaches, migraines, indigestion and poor circulation. The essential oil can soothe arthritis, rheumatism and muscular aches and pains, acts as a stimulant and painkiller, and may be used as a hair tonic to encourage growth and restore colour.

SAGE

Regular cups of sage tea were once regarded as a guarantee of long life, as the old country rhyme – "he who drinks sage in May, shall live for aye" – reminds us. The herb is believed to restore failing memory in the elderly. The red or purple variety is preferred by herbalists, but many members of the sage family possess similar properties.

Today the plant is known to be an antioxidant which can combat free radicals and cell decay. It is also rich in oestrogenic substances. Sage has an important affinity with the throat and mouth and makes an excellent gargle and mouthwash for many infections and inflammations. The leaves can be used in creams and ointments for minor cuts and insect bites. Sage is drying, and can be used by breast-feeding mothers when weaning to reduce milk production. The Chinese use the root of another variety. *Salvia miltiorrhiza* (*dan shen*) as a tonic.

INDEX

ACKNOWLEDGMENTS

The author and the publishers gratefully acknowledge the invaluable contribution made by David Jordan who took all the photographs in this book except: 16 top ; 21 middle Ia; 23 bottom Iai; 27 top Z; 33 David de Lossy/The Image Bank; 39 bottom left John Gerlach/Earth Scenes/Oxford

Also thanks to the following who kindly supplied material for photography: The Boots Company PLC; Geffrye Museum, Kingsland Road, London E2 8EA; San Ling Chinese Medicine Centre, 97b Golders Green Road, London NW11 8EN; Bennett and Luck Health Foods, 52 Islington Park Street, London N1 1RL; Neal's Yard, 15 Neals Yard, London WC2H 9DP; East West Herbs Shop, 3 Neals Yard, London WC2 9DP; Helios Homeopathic; Paula Pryke Flowers, 20 Penton Street, London N1 9PF; Chelsea Physic Garden' 66 Royal Hospital Road, London SW3 4HS; Virgo Bodywork Tables, Rowley's Yard, Woodlands Park Road, London N15 3RT